NUTRITION HANDBOOK

Dr. Bernard Jensen's
Daily Regimen for Healthy Living

For Patient Use
and Nutritional Counseling

Taken from Dr. Jensen's
Series on Kitchen Chemistry

Bernard Jensen, Ph.D.
Clinical Nutritionist

PUBLISHED BY:

Bernard Jensen, Ph.D.
24360 Old Wagon Road
Escondido, CA 92027 USA

The health procedures in this book are based on the training, personal experiences and research of the author. Because each person and situation is unique, the publisher urges the reader to check with a qualified health professional before using any procedure where there is any question as to its appropriateness.

Because there is always some risk involved, the author/publisher are not responsible for any adverse effects or consequences resulting from the use of any of the suggestions, preparations or procedures in this book. Please do not use the book if you are unwilling to assume the risk. Feel free to consult a physician or other qualified health professional. It is a sign of wisdom, not cowardice, to seek a second or third opinion.

Second Edition

BERNARD JENSEN, Publisher
24360 Old Wagon Road
Escondido, CA 92027 USA

ISBN 0-932615-30-9

Dedication

TO MY BROTHERS and SISTERS who are hungry and thirsty for all the life and energy we get from nutrition for healing and building the integrity of our cell life.

CONTENTS

INTRODUCTION

There is a good deal of confusion about foods and what is best to eat today. We should be concerned about what we are consuming. Most people have little understanding of what the body is made from. People build a body chemistry on the kinds of foods they eat. The body is as healthy as the kinds of foods it has been built from. It is the way we are living and eating that will determine our future. Self care should be an important part of our daily lives. Hippocrates said, "Let food be your medicine and your medicine by your food." He also said that the doctor of the future will never understand disease until he understands the makeup of food. Nutrition can play a vital role in rebuilding and repairing the immune system.

There is much study of non-toxic elements being done today for the health of the body. Many people who have been treated with drugs have iatrogenic illnesses. People who have been exposed to toxic chemicals are suffering from chemical illnesses. Statistics show that twenty thousand tons of aspirins are being used yearly. Forty million people in this country now have allergies. One out of three people are dying annually with cancer and nine out of ten suffer from colon disorders. It has been found that 54% of our deaths come from heart disease and 77% of the population have some form of arthritis. In addition, 58% of our children fail in fitness tests. It is my opinion that it is time for us to look for answers to these problems in correcting the lifestyle and choosing to eat organically-grown foods.

I have spent many years of research putting food ideas into an orderly manner. I have attempted to present food concepts in a simple, practical way so people can better understand how to properly nourish their bodies. Confusion about nutrition causes people to listen to repetitious commercials and be overcome by them. The worst thing about the products on the market today is that many of them are not developed by dietitians, doctors, nutritionists or people with suitable training. Last year, every man, woman and child in the U.S. spent $1,964 on health care alone. Scientific reports are telling us that a well-balanced diet enriched with fruits and vegetables, grains, low fat, low sugar and low salt, significantly lowers the risks for developing heart disease, cancer, osteoporosis, arthritis and other degenerative diseases.

A spokeswoman for the National Food Processors Association said that food labels should communicate facts and not educate. I think this is true, but I also feel that people need a nutritional program that is uncomplicated and easy to understand. Many people are asking pertinent questions about what kinds of foods are best to eat. Should we eat grains? Is meat good for us? Should we leave out milk entirely? Do we need salt?

I have developed a nutritional program that will prosper the body, feed burned out tissues, take care of damaged cell structure and repair, rebuild and rejuvenate any breakdown of tissue that may have occurred in the cell structures of the body. I have found that the mind needs certain kinds of foods. The glands need another kind of food. The bones need still another kind. If we neglect any system in the body, any organ of the body, that system or organ can become starved and have a lowered functional ability. Every organ has to be fed so it can keep functioning normally. This nutritional handbook is a simple, step-by-step, practical program I have developed over many years to help guide my patients into a healthy lifestyle and to ensure they furnish the nutritional requirements their bodies need.

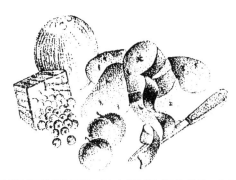

1. RECOMMENDED DAILY FOOD PROGRAM

My Food Healing Laws follow. These laws will take care of the proper calorie intake, enzymes, vitamins and minerals. Always remember the importance of foods as described in these laws. Our health is determined as much by what we don't eat as well as what we do eat, which can cause nutritional deficiencies that lead to future disease. If we neglect vegetables, for example, we prevent our bodies from receiving needed chemical elements and enzymes. Lack of sufficient proteins, carbohydrates and fats can cause disturbances in the body, as can the lack of vitamins, minerals, lecithin, enzymes and trace elements. All of these have to be considered.

I believe there are three basics that lead to disease. First are **inherent weaknesses** we have inherited from our parents. Second are the **toxic materials** we have accumulated in our bodies from pollution, chemicals, drugs or junk foods. Third are the **chemical deficiencies** we have in the body. My food program is designed to help the body overcome these weaknesses. It will help build the immune system as well as strengthen the inherent weaknesses, remove the toxic material buildup in the body and replace the needed biochemicals. The foods I have recommended will nourish the body with the needed nutrients as well as rid the body of any chemical deficiencies.

3

Law No. 1: EAT NATURAL, PURE, WHOLE AND FRESH FOODS

If you would like to be healthy and have a strong immune system consume only those foods that are **natural, pure, whole and fresh**. This means that the foods should be organic, without insecticides or sprays. They should be grown on rich soil that contains all the minerals necessary for the health of the plants as well as for the health of the human body. Foods must be whole, without added preservatives, extra salt or sugar. The spices, sauces and condiments that people use are irritating to the body. Black pepper can be very irritable to the liver. Often hypertension in children is caused by extra sugar, preservatives, food dyes and condiments in the body. Doctors are making a living on people who take excessive amounts of sugar, salt, alcohol and caffeine.

Foods high in white sugar should be avoided entirely. If one eats any sweets at all, they should come from nature, pure and whole foods. Fruits have plenty of sugar. Dried fruits, such as dates, figs, prunes and raisins make a wonderful dessert high in iron. A little raw honey or maple syrup occasionally will not hurt. Sixty years ago, we averaged 16 pounds of sugar per person in the U.S. annually. Today, Americans average 115 pounds of sugar per person each year. This is far too much.

I go into a restaurant and watch people add salt to their foods before they even taste it. If a person has used salt for years, their taste buds have become numb and they need more and more of it to be able to taste it. Athletes who sweat hard and lose as much as 10-12 pounds in a professional game may use sun-evaporated sea salt. I feel that table salt (which is sodium chloride and often contains aluminum) should be avoided entirely. Nature provides us with plenty of organic sodium in fresh vegetables and fruit. Sodium in this natural form is very necessary to our health.

Coffee, soft drinks and chocolate (which are all high in caffeine) should be eliminated from the diet completely. Caffeine is a strong stimulate to the pancreas and the liver and it has no nourishment value at all. Alcohol is very hard on the pancreas and liver as well. The body has to use many of its vital nutrients in order to process the alcohol and the alcohol gives no nutrients to the body in return. In many restaurants and bars notices are posted warning pregnant women they can harm their unborn child with alcohol. When the body is balanced with all the nutritional elements it needs to be well nourished, it will not have such a craving for denatured foods, sugar, salt, caffeine or alcohol.

There are certain foods that should be avoided because they are not whole, fresh and pure. We should avoid fried foods, foods high in fats, white rice, pasteurized milk products and white flour, which is high in gluten. Gluten causes celiac disease, which is an intestinal malabsorption syndrome characterized by diarrhea, malnutrition, bleeding tendency and hypocalcemia. Treatment of this disease is a gluten-free diet that may have to be continued for an indefinite period. Intestine villi, which are necessary for the absorption of nutrients, can be "glued together" by the pasty substance called gluten.

The average American consumes 25% of the diet in milk products. This is far too much. Milk substitutes, such as nut and seed milks, can replace cow's milk in your diet. I believe in using fresh goat's milk. Besides its pleasant taste, it is closest to human milk. It is a brain food, high in chlorine and is effective in kidney disturbances because it is germicidal in effect. I have seen the sick virtually revived from a death-bed with fresh, warm goat milk and could cite case after case where the use of goat milk has been successful in transmitting the necessary particles of nutrition to the body. This is because it is easier to digest and assimilate into the bloodstream. Goat milk is surely a vitality-producing food.

If you were to study the chemical nature of the human body, you would gain a better understanding of the importance of foods being natural, whole, fresh and pure. When the body becomes deficient in certain chemical elements, the symptoms of scurvy, beriberi or other diseases may occur. Sailors at sea discovered this many years ago, and began to take citrus fruits with them on their journeys. Often whole countries can be affected. In Denmark at one time all the butter was taken to London to feed pilots who had developed eye problems and night blindness. This was when vitamin A was discovered.

I believe there isn't a disease in which the person does not have mineral shortages and dietary deficiencies. The best way to be sure we get all the nutrients we need to be healthy is to eat foods that are as close as possible to the way nature provides them—fresh, whole, natural and pure.

Law No. 2: SIXTY PERCENT OF EVERYTHING YOU EAT SHOULD BE RAW

In my research, I have found that raw foods contain living enzymes that are magnetically attracted to the living cells in the body. Living cells can better utilize the nutrients from raw foods than from cooked foods. In addition, raw foods are higher in vitamins and minerals than foods that have been cooked. Heating often destroys the vital elements in the foods. Some nutritionists might say a person should consume 100% raw foods; however, I feel this approach is quite extreme and could be very difficult for most people to follow. I believe that 60% of the diet should be raw foods.

Reports say that eggs are high in cholesterol. However, lecithin is one of the finest things to help lower cholesterol and is found highest in the raw egg yolk. The raw egg yolk is also one of the most complete proteins one can consume. Eggs have all the nutrients necessary to build a new life. It is a wonderful food for the brain and nervous system. Raw egg yolks can be blended into black cherry juice, which makes a very wonderful drink that is high in iron and a great tonic for the nerves.

Raw seeds and nuts are also very high in protein and are excellent foods for the glands. We are becoming a "seedless generation," as markets are now carrying hybrid fruits, oranges, tangerines and even watermelons, that contain no seeds. Nuts and seeds are very helpful for men and women who are experiencing infertility problems.

Raw fruits are high in bioflavonoids, which are necessary for healthy connective tissues in the skin, veins and capillaries. Bioflavonoids can prevent wrinkles, varicose veins and hemorrhoids (which are caused by straining the tissue in the rectum).

Raw green vegetables are high in chlorophyll, which is necessary for clean, healthy blood. Chlorophyll and blood are similar in content except that blood has the red hemoglobin factor. Raw yellow vegetables are high in beta carotene, which is necessary for the immune system and has been researched to help prevent cancerous tissue from forming.

Chewing raw foods daily helps to develop good teeth, healthy gums and strong jaws. Be sure to chew your food about 32 times for each bite so you will receive all the nutrients in the food and digest it well. Eat plenty of raw vegetables, nuts, seeds and fruits from Mother Nature's bounteous table each day to build a healthy, happy body.

Law No. 3: BALANCE YOUR DIET WITH 80% ALKALINE FOODS AND 20% ACID FOODS

Eighty percent of the nutrients carried in the blood are alkaline and twenty percent are acid. To keep the blood the way it should be, I have found that 6 vegetables and two fruits make up the 80% alkaline foods we need, while 1 protein and 1 starch make up the 20% acid foods.

Proteins and many starches are acid-forming and nearly all the metabolic wastes of the body are acid. We need alkaline-forming foods such as fruit and vegetables so their alkaline salts will neutralize the acid wastes. We should recognize that the fresher the food, the more alkaline it is. The longer it is kept, the more acid it becomes.

Meats contain uric acid so should be eaten sparingly. Uric acid can cause high blood pressure, gout, arthritis, urinary tract disorders and many other problems. People who suffer from too much uric acid in the body have eaten too much meat and not enough alkaline salads. There is no reason we should add to the acid conditions in our body by including heavy acid foods such as found in proteins and starches. In my experience, acid waste not properly disposed of is the cause of many disturbances, health problems and chronic diseases.

Law No. 4: CONSUME 6 VEGETABLES, 2 FRUITS, 1 STARCH AND 1 PROTEIN DAILY

During my many years of research and working with over 300,000 patients with various nutritional deficiencies and ailments, I worked out these proportions as being the best and most beneficial for allowing the body to receive all the nutrients it needs on a daily basis. This proportion can be used for all ages; however, the diet of children can be altered to include 2 starches and 1 protein daily. For those who are over the age of 40, their diet can possibly contain 2 proteins and 1 starch daily. This may be preferable, and can be regulated according to the physical or mental expressions and activities.

Vegetables are high in fiber and minerals. Fruits are high in natural complex sugars and vitamins. Starch is for energy and protein is for cell repairing and rebuilding, especially the brain and nerves.

Remember, it is important to eat 80% of the alkaline foods daily and 20% of the acid foods daily. Six vegetables plus two fruits make up the 80% alkaline proportion. One starch plus one protein will make up the 20% acid proportion. When you eat these amounts, you will have balanced proportions of acid and alkaline foods as well as all the fiber and nutrients your body needs to be healthy.

Most nutritionists believe we should have a certain amount of carbohydrates each day, and I agree. I also believe we need a certain amount of vitamins, minerals and proteins each day, and by eating foods in the proportions I have listed, you will get all you need.

Eating a variety of vegetables is important, especially the cruciferous vegetables. Researchers have found that they are very helpful in preventing cancer. These high-sulfur foods also help to develop lecithin, which is a dissolver of hardening in the arteries and cholesterol excess. A recent review of 156 studies published in the *Journal of Nutrition and Cancer* showed that in 128 of the studies, fruits and vegetables offered significant protection against cancers of the lungs, colon, breast, cervix, esophagus, oral cavities, stomach, pancreas and ovaries. Greens are wonderful for building up the iron in the body. They are a tonic for anemics. Iron is a key component in building hemoglobin. Iron attracts oxygen, and these are the two "frisky horses" that give us energy to work with.

Calcium is found in nuts, beans, legumes, greens and grains. Children and young people need more calcium than people who are over 30 because they are building bone. Some people feel they need to get all of their calcium from milk products. We can become anemic if we eat too much heavy cream, milk, buttermilk, cheese and yogurt, because milk products are lacking in iron. These foods can also build unwanted mucus and catarrh in the body.

For the vegetables and fruits, choose those that are fresh, organically grown and vine ripened, when possible. For your daily starch requirement, choose from whole grains such as rice, rye, millet, oats, barley and yellow cornmeal. These can be cooked as a hot cereal with nut or seed milk over them.

Avoid wheat and bread. Most people have allergies to wheat because American bodies have become over saturated with it. Bread usually contains yeast and is not good for those with digestive troubles or Candida albicans.

For your protein, choose from the nuts, seeds, legumes, soft-boiled eggs, raw goat milk or cheese, organically-raised meat. One may have fish three times a week and meat once or twice a week. The king of the nuts is the almond because it is the only nut that is alkaline and high in minerals. The king of the seeds is the sesame, which is very high in calcium. The easiest to digest of the legumes is the lentil. If a person prefers to be a vegetarian, they can acquire their proteins from the nuts, seeds and legumes.

Law No. 5: EAT A VARIETY OF FOODS EVERY DAY

It is important to eat a variety of foods each day. Some people like to eat job potatoes; others like to eat only meat. When we look at the intricate chemical makeup of the body, we can see it is composed of and has the necessity for many different kinds of vitamins, minerals, enzymes, cell salts and chemical elements. Within the body is an entire universe with multitudinous functions. This is why I stress the importance of eating a wide variety of foods that are whole, pure, natural and fresh. If we eat these kinds of foods in variety, we can be more assured of getting the vital elements needed by the body to be healthy, strong and vibrant.

I feel that a healthy way of living and eating is probably the most important thing to consider. Our bodies are made from the elements of the earth, and our bones need a different food than our muscles. The adrenal gland has a different makeup than the thyroid. Our lung structure needs different foods than our eyes.

Often people do not have an adequate understanding about their bodies and nutrition. They do not understand how to incorporate a wide variety of foods on a daily basis, so they turn to diets. There are so many diets being applied to the problems that exist today. There are reducing diets, carrot juice diets, junk food diets, rice diets and protein diets. There are so many reasons why these diets have been promoted, but we find with all dietetic programs we have today, very few people actually have a healthy way of living. When people follow very limited diets, they surely have not considered the wide varieties of foods that are necessary to acquire the proper nourishment they need for every organ. We need to understand that the body needs calcium, silicon, sodium, iodine and all the other various chemical elements and trace minerals found in the earth.

There are numerous misconceptions of what makes a good food. People believe they have to be careful of calories, not realizing that one full cup of spinach contains only 14 calories and the same amount of pecan pie contains 1,000 calories! It is the **quality** of food that is important. We need a certain amount of calories to run the body properly, but the calories should come from a wide variety of foods that are pure, whole, natural and fresh. When we eat these kinds of foods, they will balance the body chemistry, the health level will improve and weight will become balanced.

If you want to lose weight, follow my healthy way of eating, and cut down all portions to a child's size for one month or longer. The amount you eat determines a good deal the weight you will have. Have 2 green vegetables a day. This is the healthy way to live and diet. This program is half eliminating and half building.

Fad diets may take the weight off for a short period of time, but this cannot last when the person returns to their old way of eating. A rice diet or a carrot juice diet *may* improve the health for a time, but if the person has not learned a new way of living and eating and they continue with the lifestyle that caused the problem in the first place, the weight is bound to return.

So, we must eat foods in a variety that are pure, nature, whole and fresh. Proper nutrition (providing all the nutrients the body needs) can help prevent atherosclerosis, heart disease and other degenerative ailments. Atherosclerosis can be produced from a lack of organic sodium, which keeps the veins and arteries soft and supply. We have to have potassium to prevent heart troubles. We need organic sodium and vitamin B-6 to keep the joints loose and limber. The pancreas needs silicon to be healthy, and the thyroid needs iodine. We must have certain foods and the nutrients contained within those foods to keep all the functions of the body working properly.

In studying color, you will find that each color has a different effect on the body. Red is an arterial stimulant. Cayenne pepper brings up the circulation and improves the digestion. Green is healing. Green foods are sedative and can help us to be more relaxed. Practically all vegetables and fruits that are considered laxative in nature are yellow and orange. This is why I teach my students to eat a "rainbow" salad filled with a variety of colorful vegetables and thus a variety of nutrients.

I have taught my students about the "sevens" in order to help them have a variety of foods each day. Know seven good salads, seven good salad dressings, seven good proteins and seven good starches. Try to work out the variety to the best of your ability and expectation and then learn more than seven; try 14, so you can improve your intake of variety.

Law No. 6: SEPARATE STARCHES AND PROTEINS

Try to separate starches and proteins if you can. The reason for this is that starches are digested by the enzyme amylase (which is alkaline), and proteins are mostly digested by hydrochloric acid, pepsin and trypsin (which are acidic). If the stomach contains both starches and proteins, both types of enzymes will be attempting to digest the food, but they do not work well together because one is alkaline and the other acidic. This can lead to indigestion, with the starches fermenting and the proteins putrefying. I don't feel that people should be fanatic about this because I have seen people not get the vitamins and minerals they need because they are working so hard on proper food combining. If a person is extremely ill or has a digestive disorder, then they need to be more careful about food combining. Separating starches and proteins assists the body in efficient digestion.

I recommend that you have your proteins and starches at different meals, not because they don't digest well together, but so you will be able to eat more fruits and vegetables at each meal. People tend to fill up on protein and starch, then neglect their vegetables. I want you to have several vegetables with each meal for your health's sake, and when you are hungry, they taste wonderful. There are poor combinations, and I will mention a few. Dried fruits do not go well with fresh fruits.

Unless dried fruits have been reconstituted and brought back to their natural state, it is best not to eat them. It is best not to have grapefruit and dates together. Dried fruits must be reconstituted by putting the dried fruit in cold water at night and bringing them to a boil, let the water boil for about 3 minutes, then turn off the flame and let them stand overnight. Melon should be eaten at least half an hour apart from any other food.

Don't have ice-cold drinks with meals because they interfere with digestion. Herb teas can be taken with meals and so can vegetable or fruit juices, since they are foods. There is much discussion about having liquids with meals. One thought is that the additional water in liquids will dilute the enzyme concentration and reduce their ability to digest the food. I believe the best source of water is from uncooked fruits and vegetables, where it has been filtered by the plant's root system. It is best to have your fruit at breakfast and at 3 pm.

One should eat a starch with a salad for a meal (for example, a salad and a baked potato) or a protein, a salad and some steamed vegetables at another meal (for example, broiled fish, salad and steamed broccoli). These menus can be used for lunch or dinner. One should always eat a raw salad with a heavy starch or with a protein in order to have the fiber and live enzymes to aid digestion.

There is possibly an age period when we need more protein and another age period when we need more starches. In the first third of our lives, when we are very active and building new tissues every day, we need more of the carbohydrates. In our later years, when we are less active physically and perhaps using our minds more, we could perhaps need more proteins. Proteins are food for the brain and nervous system. Throughout our lives, we should use wisdom in our choice of foods and combinations of foods in order to have the best possible health.

Law No. 7: INCLUDE FIBER

We have to consider fiber. There are soluble and insoluble types. Most foods have a mixture of these. We need a certain amount of fibrous material in the bowel for it to function properly. Oat bran has been known to reduce the cholesterol counts in some people. Dr. Burkitt found that the people in South Africa who had plenty of fiber in their diets, did not develop colon cancer. The people in England ate very little fiber and they were plagued with colon cancer.

The soluble fiber that is found in sprouts, cruciferous vegetables, salad vegetables and lentils can reduce the blood cholesterol levels. In an analysis of 10 clinical trials published recently in the *Journal of the American Medical Association*, it was shown that eating oat bran cereal everyday can lower blood cholesterol by 2-3 percent on the average. We also need the insoluble fibers in our intestinal tract to relieve constipation.

The National Cancer Institute recommends that Americans eat 20-35 grams of fiber a day. We are finding that whole grains, particularly flax, are high in certain compounds that can be used to develop a greater working bowel and help to overcome constipation. Cancer of the breasts has been reduced by using fiber in the diet. Blood sugar disorders, such as hypoglycemia and diabetes, have been known to improve after increasing the amount of fiber in the diet. Follow my food plan. Eat the nuts, seeds, vegetables, fruits and grains, and you will have the finest fiber in the amounts your body needs.

Law No. 8: DO NOT OVEREAT

The healthiest people I have met in my world travels were the same weight later in life as when they were in their twenties, and some of them were over 120 years of age! In the U.S., 60% of the people are overweight, which leads to many health problems. When the body is overweight, the heart has to pump harder, the circulation is slower, pressure is placed on the feet and legs, often the colon will prolapse from the extra weight, which, in turn, presses on the other organs. A person will have less energy when he is overweight and often the self esteem is lowered. Leave that extra food on the plate. Eating at home is more desirable, since restaurants often add additional oils and fats to their foods.

Overeating can cause many disturbances in the body. When the digestive tract is heavy and overburdened with foods, it becomes sluggish and slows down. This can cause constipation and a poor absorption of the nutrients we need. When the colon becomes constipated and overloaded with waste materials it cannot pass out, this begins to seep through osmosis to other parts of the body. This puts a burden on the kidneys and the skin. People with skin conditions most likely have toxic colons.

We have too many overweight people in our country. This can be caused by overeating as well as incorrect eating. In this country, 29% of the diet is made up of wheat, which builds fat. Rye builds muscle. When a person is nourished with the proper nutrients they need, and are living a happy life, then they will not need to overeat. If a person is overweight, they should not leave out the foods that are nourishing to their bodies. They should just cut out about 1/3 of all the food they are used to eating. In working with the ideal diet, we should be aware of how we take care of ourselves when we are traveling and when visiting friends. We can always choose good foods to eat. It is also a good idea to fast one day a week or eat minimal amounts. Food should never control us. We should eat only the foods that will meet our need to have a chemically-balanced body.

Some people have poor eating habits. They gorge themselves at times and starve themselves at other times. This upsets the body's metabolism. Some people do not get the nutrients they need during the meal so they binge on sugary snacks throughout the day.

There are many things that could be said about weight control. Experts are finding it is very beneficial to follow a low-fat diet. If one consumes oils, they should come from whole grains and not be heated above 212 degrees. A good, sensible way of eating, positive thinking practices and a balance of exercise will bring most people's weight to normal.

Law No. 9: COOK WITHOUT WATER, HIGH HEAT OR AIR TOUCHING HOT FOOD

High heat, boiling in water and exposure to air are the three greatest robbers of nutrients. Always cook with low temperatures. It is impossible to get the best of the nutritional values out of oils if they have been heated above 212 degrees or the boiling temperature. Lecithin is destroyed in those foods that are fried or cooked and baked in ovens that are over 212 degrees. People would not have the high cholesterol problems if they would use cold-pressed oils that have not been heated. Raw egg yolks are very high in lecithin, which dissolves cholesterol.

Low-heat stainless steel pots with lids that form a water seal are the most efficient means of cooking foods in such a way as to preserve the greatest nutritional value. For oven cooking, glass casserole dishes with lids are fine. I approve of crockpot cooking because it offers another low-heat method.

I do not approve of the microwave oven. When wheat is cooked in a microwave oven and then put into the ground, it will not grow. But if you cook wheat at low temperatures in low-heat, stainless steel cookware and put it into the ground, it will still sprout. Low-heat stainless steel cookware is very important, in my estimation, in taking care of our dietetic procedure.

Law No. 10: BAKE, BROIL, ROAST OR STEAM MEATS

Meat should be eaten sparingly—no more than three times a week. It is preferable to eat fish or chicken. If one does eat red meat, it should be no more than once a week, and should have all the fat trimmed off. Never fry meats. Fried foods are very difficult to digest due to the high-fat content. Baking, broiling, roasting or steaming are far from perfect cooking methods, but are more acceptable by preserving more nutritional values. Cook at lower heats for longer times to retain the most nutritional value.

Avoid pork and fatty meats and use only white fish with fins and scales. Salmon is permitted, even though it isn't a white meat fish. Fatty meats lead to obesity and heart trouble. Beef is very stimulating to the heart, and I do not recommend using it. Eating meat more than three times a week can produce excess uric acid and other irritating by-products causing an unnecessary burden on the body. While I do not believe that the meat will cause heart trouble, I believe when we live a fast, hard lifestyle that includes having a heavy amount of meat, it can lead to heart troubles. Those who study the positive and negative effects of food will find that meat is positive, starches are negative. Starches feed the left side of the body which is the side where the heart is located. Proteins feed the right side of the body.

Law No. 11: BE CAREFUL OF YOUR DRINKING WATER

Most public water systems are now highly chemicalized because ground water sources are increasingly polluted. The fruit and vegetables in my food regimen supply much of the water your body needs. If you use broths, juices, soups and herbal teas, they will take care of any remaining thirst during the day. If you are still thirsty, try cutting down or eliminating salt on your foods. Salt creates a thirst. Use vegetable or broth seasonings instead. I advise using distilled water for those who have arthritis. We don't really need much drinking water on my food regimen. Reverse osmosis water purification units provide the best water for household consumption.

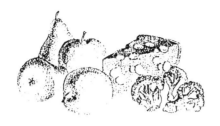

2. HEALTH-BUILDING FOODS BEGIN AT HOME

Let your food be your medicine, and your medicine be your food, is a message carved in stone and left to us by Hippocrates (460-370 B.C.), the ancient Greek healer credited with being the "father of modern medicine."

This ancient true is as valid today as it was over 2,000 years ago. Whole, raw, natural, non-chemical, unprocessed foods contain an element of health that cannot be duplicated in any other way. Time and time again, researchers have proven this fact. Animals fed on synthetic diets always die of starvation, malnutrition and deficiency diseases. The very essence of nature cure healing is founded upon this truth. Nature inherently contains all the necessary preconditions for health and vitality when left undisturbed. It is the tampering of man that upsets this balance and throws him into states of disease.

Quality food is the first line of defense and base rock foundation upon which vibrant health and well-being are built. The literature as testimony to this fact is abundant. In all cases, processing of any kind, especially the application of heat, destroys food values. There are very delicate essences present in fully-ripened food grown on rich organic soil that can only be appreciated when eaten in the fresh, raw state.

DR. JENSEN'S HEALTH AND HARMONY
FOOD REGIMEN

The best diet, over the period of a day, is 2 different fruits, at least 4-6 vegetables, 1 protein and 1 starch, with fruit or vegetable juices between meals. Eat at least 2 green leafy vegetables a day. Fifty-to-sixty percent of the food you eat daily should be raw. Dr. Jensen designed this General Diet Regimen as the result of his research with thousands of people who came to his sanitarium, where he worked and taught classes on nutrition for over 40 years. He saw many people rebuild their health and regain their strength on this program. If you will make a habit of applying the following General Diet Regimen to your everyday living, you will be pleased at how much better you will begin to feel.

Rules of Eating

1. Do not fry foods or use heated oils.
2. If not entirely comfortable in mind and body, do not eat.
3. Do not eat unless you have a keen desire for the plainest food.
4. Do not eat beyond your needs.
5. Be sure to thoroughly masticate your food.
6. Miss meals if in pain, emotionally upset, not hungry, chilled, overheated and during illness.

Rules for Getting Well

1. Learn to accept whatever decision is made.
2. Let the other person make a mistake and learn.
3. Learn to forget and forgive.
4. Be thankful and bless people.
5. Live in harmony—even if it is good for you.
6. Do not talk about your sickness.

7. Gossip will kill you. Don't let anyone gossip to you either. Gossip that comes through the grapevine is usually sour grapes!
8. Be by yourself every day for 10 minutes with the thought of how to make yourself a better person. Replace negative thoughts with uplifting, positive thoughts.
9. Skin brush daily. Use a slant board daily.
10. Exercise daily; keep your spine limber. Develop abdominal muscles. Do sniff breathing exercises. Have a daily set of exercises.
11. Grass and sand walk for happy feet.
12. No smoking or drinking alcohol.
13. Bed at sundown, 9 pm at the latest. If you are at all tired, fatigued or unable to do your work with vim and vigor, rest more. Rest more if you are ill. Sleep out of doors, out of the city, in the circulating air. Work out problems in the morning; don't take them to bed with you.

Food Healing Laws

1. Natural food: 50-60% of food eaten should be raw.
2. Your diet should be 80% alkaline and 20% acid.
3. Proportion: 6 vegetables, 2 fruits, 1 starch and 1 protein daily.
4. Variety: vary sugars, proteins, starches, vegetables and fruits from meal-to-meal and day-to-day.
5. Overeating: you can kill yourself with the amount of food you eat.
6. Combinations: separate starches and proteins. One at lunch and the other at dinner. Have fruits for breakfast and at 3 pm.
7. Cook without water; cook without high heat; cook without air touching hot food.
8. Bake, broil or roast; if you eat meat, have it but only 3 times a week. This includes poultry, fish and lean meats; no fat, no pork; red meats are not

recommended. Use non-sprayed vegetables, if possible, and eat them as soon after being picked as possible.

9. Use stainless steel low-heat cooking utensils; it is the modern health-engineered way to prepare your foods.

Before Breakfast

Upon rising and 1/2 hour before breakfast, take any natural, unsweetened fruit juice, such as grape, pineapple, prune, fig, apple or black cherry. Liquid chlorophyll can be used also; also use 1 teaspoon of vegetable broth powder and 1 tablespoon of lecithin granules and dissolve in a glass of warm water. Between fruit juice and breakfast, do the following: skin brushing, exercise, walking, hiking, deep breathing or playing. When showering, start with warm water and cool off until your breath quickens. Never shower immediately upon rising.

Breakfast

Stewed fruit, one starch and a health drink—or two fruits, one protein and a health drink. (Starches and health drinks are listed with the lung suggestions.) Soaked fruits, such as unsulfured apricots, prunes, figs. Fruit of any kind—melon, grapes, peaches, pears, berries or baked apple, which may be sprinkled with some ground nuts or nut butter. When possible, use fruit in season.

Suggested Breakfast Menus

Monday

Reconstituted dried apricots
Steel-cut oatmeal - Supplements
Oatstraw tea
Add eggs, if desired, or sliced peaches
and raw cottage cheese

Tuesday

Fresh figs
Cornmeal cereal - Supplements
Shave grass tea
Add eggs or nut butter, if desired, or
Raw applesauce and blackberries

Wednesday

Reconstituted dried peaches
Millet cereal - Supplements
Alfa-mint tea
Add eggs, raw cheese or nut butter, or
Sliced nectarines and apple and raw yogurt

Thursday

Prunes or any reconstituted dried fruit
Quinoa cereal - Supplements
Oatstraw tea, or
Grapefruit and kumquats and poached egg

Friday

Slices of fresh pineapple w/shredded coconut
Buckwheat cereal - Supplements
Dandelion coffee or Herb tea

Saturday

Muesli w/bananas and dates
Goat milk - Supplements
Dandelion coffee or Herb tea

Sunday

Cooked applesauce w/raisins
Rye grits - Supplements
Shave grass tea, or
Cantaloupe and strawberries
Raw cottage cheese

Preparation Tips

Reconstituted dried fruit. Cover with cold water, bring to a boil, remove from heat and leave to stand overnight. Raisins may just have boiling water poured over them. This kills any insects and eggs.

Whole grain cereal. To cook properly with as little heat as possible, use a double boiler or Thermos to cook your cereal.

Supplements (can be added to cereal or fruit). Sunflower seed meal, rice polishings, wheat germ, flaxseed meal (about a teaspoon of each). Even a little dulse may be sprinkled over it with chlorella powder and broth powder.

Lunch

Raw salad, or as directed, one or two starches, as listed, and a health drink. The raw vegetable salad may consist of the following: Tomatoes, lettuce (no iceberg lettuce)—use green, leafy-type such as romaine—celery, cucumber, bean sprouts, green peppers, avocado, parsley, watercress, endive, grated carrots, grated beets, onion*, cabbage*. (* indicates sulfur foods.)

Starches

Yellow cornmeal, baked potato, baked banana (or at least dead ripe), barley (a winter food), steamed brown rice or wild rice, millet (have as a cereal), banana squash or hubbard squash.

Drinks

Vegetable broth, soup, coffee substitutes, raw buttermilk, raw goat milk, oatstraw tea, alfalfa-mint tea, huckleberry tea, papaya tea or any health drink.

Suggested Lunch Menus

Monday

Vegetable salad w/tahini dressing
Baby Lima beans, baked potato
Spearmint tea

Tuesday

Raw salad plate w/humus
Steamed asparagus, steamed brown rice
Vegetable broth or herb tea

Wednesday

Raw salad plate w/guacamole dressing
Cooked green beans
Cornbread or baked hubbard squash
Sassafras tea

Thursday

Salad w/raw blue cheese dressing
Baked zucchini and okra
Corn on the cob, Ry-Krisp
Carrot juice

Friday

Green leafy salad w/olive oil, herb and lemon dressing
Baked green pepper stuffed with
eggplant, millet, herbs and tomatoes
Split pea soup or fennel tea

Saturday

Vegetable salad w/health mayonnaise dressing
Steamed turnips and turnip greens
Cornbread
Catnip tea

Sunday

Vegetable salad w/lemon tahini dressing
Vegetable-barley soup
Steamed chard, baked yams
Chamomile tea

Salad Vegetables

Use plenty of greens; choose four or five vegetables from the following: Leaf lettuce, watercress, spinach, beet leaves, parsley, alfalfa sprouts, cabbage, young chard herbs, any green leaves, cucumbers, bean sprouts, onions, green peppers, pimentos, carrots, turnips, zucchini, asparagus, celery, okra, radishes, tomatoes, garlic, chives, jicama, mushrooms, fennel, buckwheat sprouts, sunflower seed sprouts, etc.

Dr. Jensen's book, *Vibrant Health from Your Kitchen*, is a complete food guide. Tables for vitamin and mineral guidance, acid and alkaline tables—with complete instructions for perfect combinations to assure you a correct daily balance—are designed to keep you well. This book shows how to cook, prepare and serve foods healthfully, the natural food way. It is illustrated with charts and recipes.

3 pm: Health cocktail, raw vegetable juice or fruit juice or fruit.

Dinner

Raw salad, two cooked vegetables, one protein and a broth or health drink, if desired.

Cooked Vegetables

Peas, artichokes, carrots, beets, turnips, string beans, Swiss chard, eggplant, zucchini, summer squash, broccoli, cauliflower, cabbage, sprouts, onion or any vegetable other than potatoes.

Drinks

Herbal teas, vegetable broth, soup, raw vegetable juices (carrot, celery, parsley, beet, fennel—any combination.

Proteins

Once a Week: Fish—use white fish, such as sole, halibut, trout or sea trout. Egg omelet.
Twice a Week: Raw cottage cheese or any cheese that breaks.
Three Times a Week: Meat—use only lean meat; never pork, fats or cured meats. Vegetarians: Use meat substitutes, vegetarian proteins or tofu.
If you have a protein at dinner, a health dessert is allowed. Never eat protein and starches together. Note how they are separated in this program.
You may exchange your noon meal for the evening meal, but follow the same regimen. It takes exercise to handle raw food, and we generally get more after our noon meal. That is why a raw salad is advised at noon. If one eats sandwiches, have vegetables at the same time.

Vegetarians

Use soybeans, lima beans, pinto beans and other beans; sunflower and other seeds, nut and seed butters, nut milk drinks, raw cheeses that break, eggs and tofu. Vegetarians must be aware that being a vegetarian is more than just a diet of cutting out meat. Dr. Jensen believes that being a vegetarian is a way of thinking and a way of life. Vegetarians can choose from the vegetarian foods listed in this program. They can also read Dr. Jensen's upcoming new set of *Kitchen Chemistry* books.

Suggested Dinner Menus

Monday

Salad
Diced celery and carrots, steamed spinach
Puffy omelet

Tuesday

Salad
Cooked beet tops
Broiled steak or ground beef patties w/tomato sauce
Cauliflower
Comfrey tea

Wednesday

Raw cottage cheese, cheese sticks
Apples, peaches, grapes, nuts
Apple concentrate cocktail

Thursday

Salad
Steamed chard, baked eggplant
Grilled liver and onions
Persimmon whip (optional)

Friday

Salad
Raw yogurt and lemon dressing
Steamed mixed greens; beets
Steamed fish w/lemon slices
Leek soup; lemon grass tea

Saturday

Salad
Cooked string beans; baked summer squash
Carrot load; lentil soup or almond tea
Fresh peach gelatin w/almond nut cream

Sunday

Salad
Diced steamed carrots and peas; tomato aspic
Roast leg of lamb w/mint sauce
Apple tea

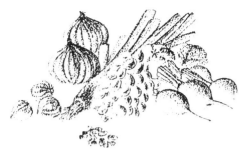

3. SPECIAL HEALTH-BUILDING FOODS

The human body is a complex structure of billions of specialized parts and electrochemical processes, constantly moving, flowing, changing, in the state of dynamic equilibrium we call life. The average lifetime of a red blood cell is 120 days, and when it dies, it is replaced by new ones. As long as we provide the body with the biochemical nutrients it needs, the various organs and tissues can rejuvenate themselves indefinitely—provided we eat the foods which contain the vitamins and minerals we need.

If the body is not given the biochemical nutrients it needs, cells break down and die before their appointed time. If it is given substances it can't digest, use or completely excrete, they remain in the body as toxic settlements in the tissue, reducing the ability of some organ or tissue structure to do its job. We must have the right foods to build and sustain high-level wellness.

I have spent over 60 years searching for the keys to good health and long life, traveling throughout the world looking for vital health secrets. I have spent many years in sanitarium work, observing first-hand what foods and therapies did for patients with varying health problems.

In my work, I often found that my patients had deficiencies in important vital chemical elements—particularly sodium, calcium, silicon and iodine. Each recipe given here was developed for the specific purpose of replacing certain nutrients that might be lacking in the body in order to assist the body in rebuilding and repairing weakened or damaged tissues. The following are special health-building recipes that I have used with great success throughout the years.

BROTH RECIPES

Potato Peeling Broth

Potato peeling broth and Whex, a dehydrated goat milk whey product, are high in organic sodium and potassium, which assist in restoring calcium balance in the body. These foods are particularly useful in bringing calcium back into solution in cases of arthritis and in taking care of sodium deficiency in underactive digestive systems.

Potato Peeling Broth Recipe

Peel 2 medium potatoes (1/4" thick) and simmer peelings only in a pint of water for 15 minutes. Strain and drink only the broth. This is a potent broth for assisting elimination. You may want to try a more varied, but equally-potent recipe as follows:

2 cups potato peelings
2 cups celery tops
1 tbsp vegetable
  broth powder

2 cups carrot tops
1 medium onion
2 qt water

Finely chop all ingredients, add to water, bring slowly to a boil; simmer 20 minutes. Strain off broth and drink one or two cups a day.

Veal Joint Broth

Sodium, which occurs naturally in certain foods, is an element I have used most successful in dealing with so many people who were suffering from arthritis and general acid conditions. Doctors measure a patient's age by the suppleness of the joints, and suppleness is attributable to sodium, the "youth element," which keeps us youthful, pliable, limber and active. Sodium's importance is widespread in the body. It keeps calcium and magnesium in solution, and is active in the lymph and blood. Lack of organic sodium can result in hardening, stiffness, rheumatism, gout and gallstones. Veal joint broth is rich in sodium and excellent for glands, stomach, ligaments and digestive disorders, as well as helping to retain youth in the body.

Veal Joint Broth Recipe

Wash a fresh, uncut veal joint, and put into a large cooking pot; cover half with water and add the following vegetables and greens, cut finely:

Small stalk of celery	1/2 cup parsley
1-1/2 cups apple peelings, 1/2" thick	2 cups potato peelings, 1/2" thick
2 beets, grated	1 large parsnip
1/2 cup fresh/frozen okra or 1 tsp powdered okra	1 onion

Simmer all ingredients 4-5 hours. Strain off liquid and discard solid ingredients. There should be about 1-1/2 quarts of liquid. Drink hot or warm. Keep refrigerated.

Special Broth

This is a recipe I developed specifically for those suffering with arthritis or arteriosclerosis. Whex, a commercial powdered goat whey, is high in sodium which helps to keep joints and arteries loose and limber. The broth powder helps this drink taste delicious because it is made of a variety of dried vegetables, such as celery, tomato, pimento, parsley, alfalfa, spinach, watercress and carrots. All of these vegetables contain organic sodium as well. The third item in this recipe is lecithin, which is a dissolver. Lecithin helps to dissolve hardened deposits in the veins, arteries and joints.

Special Broth Recipe

1 tsp Whex	1 tbsp lecithin granules
1 cup hot water	1 tsp vegetable broth powder

MILK SUBSTITUTE DRINKS
(Non-Catarrh Forming)

What can we use in place of milk? When we have taken such a high intake of milk into the body over the years, especially while we have been growing up and forming the different systems in our body, it is necessary we realize that having 25% milk (and milk products in our diet) is crowding out the other lovely foods we should be having. It is equally important that we find a substitute for milk, and I have found a wonderful substitute in the seed and nut milk drinks.

For all mucus and catarrhal troubles, I suggest that people eliminate wheat, milk, sugar, fats and salt from their diets. These foods often produce extra mucus in the body which can be the basis for colds, flu, bronchial trouble, allergies of all kinds, pneumonia, hay fever, sinus infections and asthma. Children and adults with serious catarrhal problems do extremely well, and a noticeable improvement in catarrhal conditions can be seen in a matter of weeks by giving up wheat and milk and by using these alternative drinks made from seed butters, sesame seeds especially, and also almond nut butter. Sunflower seeds make very good butters also. These drinks cannot develop catarrh. They make wonderful milk substitutes. You do not have to worry about the balance of chemical elements. All the calcium and growth elements are there that are necessary for a child to build a good body.

Sesame Seed Milk

2 cups water   1/4 cup sesame seeds
2 tbsp soy milk powder

Blend until smooth. Strain, if desired, to remove hulls. Variation: 1 tbsp carob powder and 6-8 dates. Blend for flavor and added nutritional value any one of the following: Banana, date powder, stewed raisins or grape sugar. After any addition, always blend to mix. This drink can also be made from goat's milk in place of the water.

I believe that sesame seed milk is one of our best. It is a wonderful drink for gaining weight and for lubricating the intestinal tract. Its nutritional value is beyond compare, as it is high in protein and minerals. This is the seed used so much as a basic food in Arabia and East India.

Other Uses for Sesame Seed Milk

Salad dressing base (recipe follows); add to fruits, after-school snacks, add to vegetable broth, use on cereals for breakfast, mix with any nut butter, take twice daily with bananas to gain weight, add to whey drinks to adjust intestinal sluggishness and with supplements such as flaxseed or rice polishings.

Sesame Seed Salad Dressing

1/2 cup raw organic sesame seed   1/2 tsp vegetable broth
   butter   seasoning
2/3-1 cup water   1/4 tsp basil
1/4 tsp dill   1/4 tsp thyme
Blend until smooth. Serve as a dip (with less water) or a dressing (more water); lemon may be added to taste.

Almond Nut Milk

Use blanched or unblanched almonds (or other nuts). Soak overnight in pineapple juice, apple juice or honey water. This softens the nut meats. Then put 3 ounces of soaked nuts into 5 ounces of water and blend for 2-3 minutes. Flavor with honey, any kind of fruit: strawberry juice, carob flour, dates or bananas. Any of the vegetable juices are also good with nut milks.

Nut milks can also be used with soups and vegetarian roasts as a flavoring or put over cereals. Almond milk is a very alkaline drink, high in protein and easy to assimilate and absorb.

Soy Milk

Soy milk powder is available in every health food store. Add 2-4 tbsp of soy milk powder to one pint of water. Sweeten with raw sugar, honey or molasses and add a pinch of vegetable seasoning. For flavor, you can add any kind of fruit, carob powder, dates and bananas.

Keep in refrigerator. Use this milk in any recipe as you would regular cow's milk. It closely resembles the taste and composition of cow's milk and will sour just as quickly, so it should not be made too far ahead of planned use.

Pumpkin, Sesame or Sunflower Seed Milk
(The vegetarian's best protein—seeds)

The same principle as used for making nut milks can be employed to make seed milks. Soak overnight, liquefy, add flavorings. Use in the diet the same as the almond nut milk. It is best to use whole seeds and blend them yourself. However, if you do not have a blender, the seed meal can be used. Seeds and nuts can be ground in an electric coffee mill. Use any seeds and nuts except peanuts. For salad dressings, use the same process, but add less water.

NUT AND SEED BUTTERS

The blender will chop nuts in 3-5 seconds, grind them to a powder in a little more time or reduce them to a butter. Quick switches to on and off at high speed, and a rubber spatula to scrape off the sides accomplish this. The longer you blend, the finer the butter.

Sesame seed butter can be purchased in a health food store in a raw organic form. If you desire to make it, you can grind the seeds in a coffee mill until they are very fine and add a small amount of sesame oil. Dry, powdered herbs such as basil, dill and thyme can be added for seasoning. Almond butter can be made in the same way by adding almond oil instead of sesame oil. If one has a Champion juicer, directions are given by them for making nut butters.

GELATIN

Gelatin is 48% calcium which is made from the joint material of bones. In Europe, people often use bones with no meat on them as a base for soups. They would cook them slowly so the gelatin would come out into the soup and then they would remove the bones. Meats contain uric acid, but gelatin contains no uric acid. This is the reason Dr. Jensen does not believe in using meat in soups. However, the gelatin from the bones is very high in organic sodium (which holds calcium in solution and can prevent arthritis).

We are as young as our joints. When the joints begin to get hard and stiff, they say you are getting old. Gelatin not only contains the sodium that holds calcium in solution and reduces stiffness, but it also contains one of the most easily absorbable forms of calcium one can put into the body. Calcium is called "the knitter" and helps to keep our bones and teeth strong.

Gelatin Recipes

Gelatin Mold

1 tbsp gelatin   1 tsp broth seasoning
2 cup tomato juice
    Dissolve the vegetable broth seasoning in 1 tablespoon cold water and gelatin. Bring the tomato juice to a boil, and add gelatin mixture, stirring well to dissolve gelatin. Pour into cups and let stand in refrigerator until set. To reduce: Always eat 1 cup of this gelatin before each meal.

Powdered Skim Milk Gelatin Mold

1/2 cup cold water   1/2 cup powdered skim milk
1 cup boiling water   1 tbsp plain gelatin or
1 tsp pure vanilla   1 tbsp agar agar
    Mix milk powder, gelatin or agar agar in 1/2 cup cold water to a smooth paste. Gradually add boiling water to dissolve. Flavor with vanilla. Pour into cups and let stand in refrigerator until set.

Apricot Pie

1 C pulped apricots, fresh   1 tbsp gelatin
  or soaked dried   3 eggs
1/3 cup lemon juice   1 cup cottage cheese
1/2 cup raw sugar   9" baked pie shell
    Mix apricots with gelatin in saucepan. Beat egg yolks, add to apricots. Heat to boiling over low heat. Cook 2 minutes, stirring occasionally. Cool to lukewarm. Add lemon juice and cottage cheese. Chill until mixture begins to thicken. Beat egg whites until stiff. Add sugar. Continue beating until sugar dissolves. Fold into apricot mixture. Pour into shell. Chill until firm.

Pumpkin Pie

1 tbsp gelatin	1 cup cold water
1 cup boiling water	1/2 tsp ginger
1 tsp vegetable salt (scant)	2 tsp cinnamon (scant)
2 cup pumpkin, stewed, sieved	Brown sugar to sweeten

Soften gelatin in cold water. Add boiling water and stir. Add remaining ingredients. Pour into graham cracker pie shell and chill in refrigerator.

Graham Cracker Crust

Pour a little melted butter in the bottom of a dish. Add crushed graham crackers and brown sugar to sweeten. Press to fit dish. Spoon pie filling over this. Chill in refrigerator.

Vanilla Ice Cream

1 cup soy milk	1 egg
1-1/4 tsp gelatin	1/3 cup honey

Blend on fast speed in liquefier until thoroughly mixed. Pour into saucepan and cook over boiling water until milk makes a white foam around edge of pan and gelatin dissolves. Cook 2 minutes longer. Return to blender. Add:

1 cup whipping cream   1-1/2 tsp pure vanilla

Mix on fast speed until blended. Freeze to a soft-mush stage. Blend again until light and creamy. Refreeze until firm enough to serve.

Peach Cream

1 cup cold milk	1 cup sesame seed milk
1/2 cup health ice cream	1 cup sliced peaches
1/4 tsp cinnamon	1 tbsp gelatin

Blend ingredients in liquefier with a few pieces of crushed ice until smooth.

Sarah's Delight

5-6 comfrey leaves   1 cup unsweetened pineapple
1 tbsp gelatin   juice
1 tbsp cold water
    Soften gelatin in cold water. Melt over boiling water.
Liquefy all ingredients until comfrey is very fine. Pour into
mold. Set. Turn out onto bed of bronze lettuce. Ring around
with shredded carrot. Garnish with a spoonful of cream dressing
and half an olive.

Cheese Cake

1 tbsp gelatin   1 lemon
1/2 cup cold water   Honey, to sweeten
1 cup boiling water   1 pint cottage cheese
    Melt gelatin in cold water, add boiling water and stir to
dissolve. Add juice and rind of lemon, honey and cottage cheese
and mix well. (Sieve cottage cheese before adding.) Spoon
mixture over graham cracker pie shell and refrigerate.

Corn Aspic

1-1/2 cup corn   1 tbsp gelatin
2 cup milk   2 tbsp cold water
1 slice onion   1/4 cup parsley
1 tsp vegetable seasoning   Paprika
    Blend corn, milk, onion, vegetable seasoning and dash of
paprika in liquefier until very smooth. (Sieve to remove hulls, if
desired.) Dissolve gelatin in cold water. Heat over boiling water
to melt. Add to corn mixture and blend. Add parsley and blend
until parsley is just chopped. Pour into mold and refrigerate.
Serve on shredded lettuce with sliced tomato garnish.

Beet Mold

2 cup sliced raw beets   1/4 cup lemon juice
1/2 cup raw sugar   2 tbsp gelatin
1/4 cup cider vinegar   1/2 cup water
1 tsp vegetable seasoning
    Mix sugar, vinegar, vegetable seasoning and water. Pour over sliced beets and steam until tender. Dissolve gelatin in lemon juice. Add hot juice from beets. Place beets in mold and pour juice over. When set, serve on endive and garnish with sliced avocado and hard-boiled eggs.

Golden Pineapple Dessert

1 tbsp gelatin   1 can crushed unsweetened
1 cup boiling water   pineapple
1/2 cup raw sugar   1 cup grated carrot
1/2 lemon (juice)   1/2 cup chopped cashews
    Melt gelatin in a little cold water, add boiling water to dissolve. Stir in sugar, add pineapple, grated carrot, chopped nuts and lemon juice. Place in refrigerator to set. Serve with honey-whipped cream.

JUICES

    Everyone should have some raw vegetable and fruit juice each day. Pomegranate juice is the greatest juice for cleansing the genitourinary tract. It can be very beneficial for bladder infections. There are many good juices such as papaya juice, mango juice and apple juice. Black cherry juice is very high in iron and one of the best juices for cleansing and nourishing the liver.
    Beet juice is beneficial to the pancreas as well as the liver and gallbladder. Experiments were made in Switzerland that showed that beet juice could regress cancer in the bodies of

rats. Beet juice assists the flow of bile from the liver and aids digestion.

Carrot juice is high in beta carotene which is particularly good for the eyes. It assists the body in building the melanin in the skin which protects us from harmful ultra-violet rays. Parsley juice is high in chlorophyll which cleanses and builds the blood. Celery juice is high in organic sodium which helps keep calcium in solution. These last three juices can be drunk separately, as well as mixed together. When we combine them, we receive more of a variety of vitamins and minerals.

Remember that variety is recommended in all menus and exercises, as well. Let us have a variety in the salad dressings, soups, juices, vegetables and fruits that we have every day. Every fruit and vegetable has its own healing factors. They are grown in different soils which contain different minerals. In getting a variety, we can be more assured of getting all of the chemical elements the body needs.

For more complete information on the health benefits from juice, wonderful juice combination recipes, juices for babies and children, read Dr. Jensen's book *Juicing Therapy*.

HERBAL TEAS

Any of the herbal teas are very helpful in a right-living regimen. Think of their value and try to relate them to the particular problem you have. For instance, for weak kidneys, there is no reason why you should not use shave grass tea, parsley tea or the kidney-bladder teas.

A good eliminating tea for kidney structure is made from juniper berries. Mash them, pour a cup of hot water over them and let stand until the boiling water is just slightly warm; drink this excellent tea for wonderful results. You may add a little honey, if you wish. Using this three times in 24 hours makes this a wonderful kidney detoxifier. You can also cook some fresh asparagus in water and take a half teacup of the water three times a day.

Peppermint tea is good for stomach trouble, as is camomile tea.

If you have lung catarrh, comfrey, mullein, echinacea and fenugreek teas may be used two or three times daily.

Flaxseed tea, for eliminating toxic materials in the bowel, is one of the great elimination and healing factors for the bowel. It is found useful for inflammation or irritations of the bowel, as well as for stomach ulcers. Flaxseed can be simmered in water for a few minutes and allowed to cool slightly before drinking. Flaxseed tea also makes an excellent soothing enema for an irritated bowel.

Oat straw tea is very high in silicon which is excellent for the skin, hair, fingernails and nerves. Oat straw tea is one tea that must be boiled over a low heat for 20 minutes.

For further information on herbs and their applications, refer to Dr. Jensen's book *Herbs: Wonder Healers.*

Herbal Teas or Tinctures

Oat Straw Tea. Oat straw tea is one of the highest foods in silicon. In my clinical experience, I found that oat straw tea helped to regenerate and strengthen the nervous system, rid the lungs of catarrh and keep the joints flexible. Its silicon content improves the hair, skin and nails. It would be beneficial for a person with a weak constitution who has weak tendons, muscles and ligaments to drink oat straw tea. Silicon has been called the magnetic element and is one of the great builders of the body. A spirited horse with a beautiful sheen to its coat has been fed a lot of silicon. Silicon helps us to feel energetic and alive. It helps our minds to work quickly.

Oat straw tea can even be used as a base for soups or cooked cereal grains. It is delicious and so good for you.

Alfalfa-Mint Tea. This is a good tea that should be on everybody's shelf. Alfalfa is the highest alkaline tea there is. Many people have over-acid bodies and this tea helps them to come into balance. The roots of alfalfa go as much as 250 feet into the ground where they collect all of the minerals the earth has to offer.

Mint helps dispel gas from the bowel and is an excellent digestive aid.

When I was in the Hunza Valley, the king invited me to his home and asked how he could get rid of his bowel troubles. I noticed that the king drank many cups of black tea daily with a good amount of sugar. I went out into the garden where I found and picked fresh alfalfa and peppermint. I took this into the kitchen and made a lovely tea. I told the king to drink this in place of the black tea. The king did and liked the new tea even better than the old one, and within one week, the king's bowel troubles improved greatly.

Hawthorne Berry Tea. This tea is high in the flavonoids and B vitamins. It is excellent for the circulation. It has often been used to restore the heart muscle wall as well as to lower cholesterol levels. It has been used successfully to treat heart disease, sore throat and skin sores. It can be beneficial in relieving diarrhea and abdominal distension. Most people who are sick have poor circulation and fatigue. All sickness is a sign of stagnation in which the blood is not getting to all of the organs and tissues as it should, and, therefore, not carrying the nutrients to the areas in the body where they need to go. Hawthorne berry tea is very beneficial to one who is ill because it supports the heart and improves the circulation so the blood can carry oxygen (which gives energy) and other important chemical elements to all parts of the body.

KB-11 Tea (Kidney/Bladder). KB-11 is a tea made from 11 different herbs that are beneficial to the kidneys and bladder. These herbs help to strengthen and cleanse the kidneys and bladder as well as help them to release excess water. It is better to drink small amounts of this tea and not overdo.

FOOD CONSIDERATIONS

- Reduce dairy product use. This includes: milk, cheese, butter, cream. Eliminate pasteurized dairy products. Use see and nut milks and nut butters instead.
- Eliminate or reduce all **processed** sugar and other processed sweeteners such as corn syrup from your diet. Use substitute sweeteners **sparingly** such as whole, raw honey, blackstrap molasses, maple syrup, rice bran syrup.
- Increase the consumption of vegetables, green, leafy vegetables and fresh fruit.
- Eliminate all caffeine-containing foods or beverages such as coffee, sodas, black teas, chocolate, etc.
- Drink at least 4 glasses of liquid each day in the form of water, juice, herb tea, etc.
- Eliminate table salt from your diet. Substitute sea salt, dulse, broth powder, vegetable seasonings, herbs.
- Substitute brown rice, millet, rye and yellow cornmeal for wheat. Cut down on starches and sugars.
- Use Sun Chlorella tablets or powder regularly to cleanse the body of heavy metals and environmental pollutants.

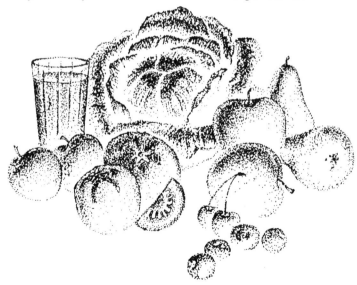

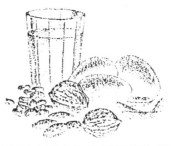

4. WHOLE FOODS WITH SEEDS

This is probably one of the most important topics in food concepts. Nuts and seeds are the beginning of the the next generation, and they are the foods of the future. Nature would not have the opportunity to carry on with a new generation without the procreative concepts found in our mineral elements, enzymes, vitamins and magnetic qualities. Seeds carry the universal life force, and nature does a very good job of putting these things together for us.

We know that seeds contain the embryo with its protective coat and stored food that can develop into a new plant under the proper conditions. Seeds take on everything possible from the mother plant. Very little air can penetrate the seed protective coat. In fact, seeds buried in King Tut's tomb 2,000 years ago were removed, planted and plants have grown. Flower seeds 200 years old were removed from the missions in Florida, planted and beautiful flowers were grown. Seeds are very important to us. When seeds from wheat and other grains are cooked in a microwave oven, they will not grow. The life force is destroyed forever.

Doctors have found there are a few mineral elements in the ground, even trace minerals, but they haven't gone so far as to find out what magnetic qualities they contain, what they need to live with one another and what is necessary to have a full complement of all the chemical elements necessary so the seeds can be grown and be whole. This means whole-minded, magnetic-minded, mineral-minded and whole trace mineral-minded, including all those things that develop an

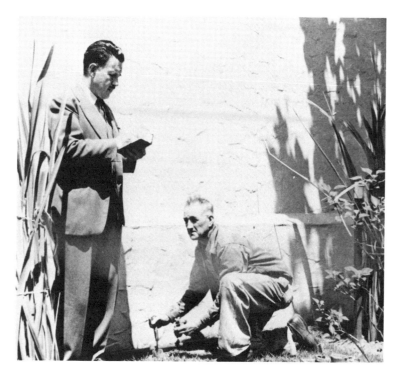

This picture shows the planting of seeds found in King Tut's tomb. They are 2,000 years old. Some were planted and they grew! It's that "life factor" in the foods we need—even today. We must have "live" foods.

electromagnetic spark ready to grow grass without it being planted from seed. All we need do is give it water, and the sunshine, air and trace minerals all work together to grow grass without first planting seed.

PROCREATION CENTER

The procreation center is found originally in the seeds and finally transformed to be used in man. There is a connection working together that makes the seeds perfect to develop the next generation. The seeds leave the mother and are ready to be planted, but they must have everything they need to begin the next generation. It is this procreative principle that is needed for the next generation's growth. They grow and develop a root structure, stems and leaves. Limbs and stems, leaves, fruit, all carry a different type of chemical makeup. A lot of this has never been studied, as far as doctors are concerned. Science is very crude in finding the finer forces in nature. Science hasn't done too good a job in finding out what nature really is, and where the real spark of life is that goes on to give the next generation its first shove and its first reproductive ability. This procreative activity is also needed for reproduction and regeneration of new cell activity when healing and correcting poorly mineralized tissue.

The root structure is dependent upon the root structure inherited from the parents, and from there, they do the best they can from what they have received. They start building a stem, building a tree with limbs, leaves, flowers and seeds that man uses for the building of his own glandular system, which will be used for developing his next generation.

There's something we have to remember. Nature is very coveteous in taking care of the seeds. She put a protective coating on nuts and seeds that cannot be penetrated. Even with the strongest digestive system, the strongest hydrochloric acid content, we cannot break down the seed covering what nature puts on almonds, sesame seeds and many other nuts and seeds.

It is well sometimes to soak these nuts and seeds overnight to breakdown the coatings, and that's why we have to liquefy, blend and break that coating down in order to make digestion easier. Eighty percent of people after the age of 50 lack hydrochloric acid. That's why health food stores and pharmacists sell so many digestive aids these days.

So it is important these foods are prepared properly in order to get the good from them into the bloodstream to repair, rebuild and re-spark the efforts in the activity of the different cell structures in the body. We should know it is not what we eat, swallow, breathe in without chewing, but what we assimilate and absorb that really counts.

The whole seed is really where the meat of our life is contained. We must get to the heart of the seed, inside the hull, and it has to be broken down in such a way that our digestive juices can make a liquid out of it so our digestive juices along the intestinal tract can get to it, break it down, change it, get it ready for the bloodstream to be delivered as a food preparation for the regeneration of cells. The body's cells must continually be regenerated. There's no part of our body that isn't visited by our blood, and our blood is only as good as the whole seeds we take into the body. The whole seed is really where the beginning of life starts, where the new cell structure begins. This is the procreation center. Seeds are the most important foods we can take into our body.

I believe the worst problem we have in this day is not educating the family cook properly. Heat breaks up the molecular balance in a lot of our foods. We began cooking by boiling water, which was all man did early on, but now we fry foods with high heat. Food material is no longer "food" because of cooking. The cooking of food with high heat, especially frying in fats and oils, causes more cholesterol problems than anything I can mention. One of the greatest of all technologies today is to strive to overcome this particular sin of civilization.

Food is destroyed with high heat. It breaks up the natural enzymes man should have to promote digestion. The natural enzymes help every other chemical element to put themselves in proper order, proper synthesization—one element with the other, to help the trace minerals in the body that are inert, and to give it the spark of life that allows a seed to grow. It's not just the mineral element factor. There is also a growth principle. Without enzymes, we will not have the new cell production we need. Enzyme therapy will be the greatest technology ever brought to man. The way we cook our foods today disturbs the molecular balance found in the natural, pure, whole, fresh foods we get from God's garden. This is the most important thing I can tell you.

To have the finest family and the best of children, those who have the best start should think about this concept. If we are going to get away from raising doctor bills we have to give the child the best health possible. It is from the seed that we raise good children.

The blood-making organs, the digestive system, are built from many forms of nutrients. Among the most important are calcium, silicon, sodium and iodine. Seed foods are filled with these minerals which help to grow a new plant. I was made aware of this while traveling through the Hunza Valley and staying with the King. There is a wonderful reflection from the mountains in the Hunza Valley. The mountains are green with mineral elements. The green represents a good production of copper in those minerals. Copper wasn't considered too important up to just a few years ago, when researchers at the University of California found that copper was very important in building a good bloodstream. We become anemic without copper in the blood. The highest amount of copper appears in apricots. This is what the Hunza people grew, and they were reaping fruit and new seeds from the same family of apricot trees for over 200 years! Isn't this amazing? This was so in the Hunza Valley because they had good seeds to produce new trees and fruit. Yes, there were 50,000 people in this community with few exceptions.

Even the apricot seed has been considered very important. It is claimed to have a direct effect on some of our most chronic and most degenerative diseases of today. But the apricot seeds had to come from a good tree. The Hunza people were free of disease. They ate the inner seed of the apricot. They even sold or traded it on the streets. It was part of their food supply, and this community that was absolutely free of disease—had no cancer, no sickness, no hospitals, no mental hospitals, no doctors, no nurses—not even a jail! They had their health because of the seed effects. This is something to think about for our future.

Most seeds or foods that have seeds, are good to eat. It is where we have the lecithin, brain and nerve foods, and where we have the regeneration principles well established. We must have the new generation and the regeneration principles from the gland foods. These gland foods allow the generations to come forth and to be in the best of health.

There are some foods with seeds we don't know too much about yet. Leave them out of your regimen. For instance, we don't know much about eating avocado seeds or peach seeds, but we do know they have effects. During World War I, peach seeds were cracked, the inner seed removed and it was used to filter out the gases used to kill soldiers.

We should have more investigation into this. We have mentioned only a partial list of the known edible seeds, but let me mention one more point that is very, very important. Only a few years ago, we couldn't even buy vitamin E. It was used in so many forms there wasn't any left for the stores to sell. Where does vitamin E come from? It's not in the flesh of the fruit—it's in the seeds. It is the procreative element that allows the seed to grow for the next generation. Without vitamin E, there is no growth in the seeds. And, around the vitamin E, is lecithin, a brain and nerve fat that feeds the glandular system and the brain and nervous system. We cannot survive without these seeds. We cannot live without vitamin E. We cannot survive without lecithin, the brain and nerve fat. And we can only get it from the seeds. This is very important.

I'm sure you understand what hybrid means, "the offspring produced by crossing two individuals of unlike genetic constitution, such as different animals or different plants." I believe this is the reason for all the glandular problems in our civilization today. We cannot build a good glandular system or regeneration system in ourselves or our plants without producing weak genes and inherent weaknesses. Originally, the orange had a hundred seeds when it was about the size of a berry, in its original state. But it was such a nuisance eating something with so many seeds! So the seeds were removed, and with that action, so were the properties to go on to provide the proper nutrients necessary for regeneration of life. They can grow oranges with extra pulp and juice, but without the glandular foundation that comes from the seeds, we are not going to grow and have the best food possible, and the glandular system of the human body will be lacking in essential nutrients and the balance of these minerals.

Some seeds contain the natural estrogen and testosterone, the female and male hormones we humans need. Some seeds have more male hormones and others have more female hormones. Citrus fruit seeds have both male and female hormones, but are higher in the female, while date seeds are very high in the male hormones. How many people know this? The Covalda Date Company started breaking down the date seed and producing it in a powdered form so it could be used along with dried dates or sprinkling on other foods. This brought some of the male hormones to the dinner table.

How many people eat citrus seeds? As I mentioned, citrus seeds contain both male and female hormones. Everyone needs male hormones, even females. And men need some female hormones also. He gets a hormonal balance in his own body by having both hormones. These are found in the seeds we consume. This is one reason we have so much trouble today not knowing if we are male or female. Mae West, one of my early patients, said it best when she said, "It's not the men in my life that counts; it's the life in my men that counts!" This is said a little crudely, but it is so true. Our strength in our generation and regeneration is found in our procreative ability we get only from the seed foods. We are starving for them, and that's why we have become a sexless generation. All the pornography and sex problems man has to deal with today are because he is not a balanced sex person in the first place.

We are producing many hybrid conditions in the human being today. We are bringing children into this world that are

50

deprived of the proper chemical elements. This would not be so if we spent more time recognizing what nature has for us. For instance, in many of the Mongoloid children born, the mother did not have enough iodine to give to the fetus. Calcium and iron are lacking in many mothers of children born today with birth defects. Doctors recognize this but it hasn't been studied enough or worked out properly. They are so busy with transplant operations, replacing wornout organs that have not been properly fed, that we are amiss in taking care of the body from a preventive standpoint rather than just trying to "fix up" problems.

Our children being born these days have chemical shortages. This means there will be still more problems in the future. We have a breakdown of certain trace minerals in the body. Unhealthy human beings are being born. You've seen notices in restaurants alerting pregnant women to the fact that alcoholic beverages may cause birth defects. Yet our polls show that many pregnant women still drink alcohol and still smoke cigarettes. Try to bring right-living methods to the average person, and it is so automatically opposed. It is unbelievable!

We are not taught how to take on some of the nicer things in life. When I lecture to my students, I ask if they deserve the right things, and they all feel they do. But why don't we take the best there is? Shame on the doctors who haven't told the people what's the very best for their good health. Health is not everything, but without it, everything else is nothing.

I am in the process now of completing a new 5-book set encyclopedia called **Kitchen Chemistry and the Mineral Body** that are books every mother, wife, cook, kitchen manager and chef should read before they prepare foods. So many foods are being destroyed through preservatives, processing, frying, overcooking, canning in aluminum, the "5 sins of civilization," which are wheat, milk, sugar, salt and fat. By gaining the proper knowledge we need in food preparation, we can be healthier, happy people.

Following are lists of seed foods that build strong bodies. While we have given only a partial list here of the whole foods with seeds, it is far from complete, and there may be many more to come in the future.

Whole Foods with Seeds

Guava	Sesame seeds	Pomegranates
Persimmons	Sunflower seeds	Almonds
Macadamias	Black walnuts	English walnuts
Pumpkins	Brazil nuts	Squash
Kiwi	Pine nuts	Watermelon
Hazel nuts	Cantaloupe	Hickory nuts
Muskmelon	Chia seeds	Honeydew
Coriander	Coconut	Loganberries
Flax seeds	Raspberries	Cod roe
Blackberries	Egg yolk	Mulberries
Strawberries	Pineapple	Blueberries
Pistachio nuts	Papaya seeds	Eggs
Quince	Figs	Okra
Beans	Prickly pears	Radishes
Cucumbers	Kumquat	and others

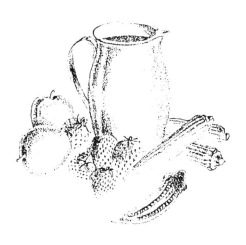

WHOLE FOODS

Whole foods have all the ability to reproduce their kind. Nature provides within the whole foods and seeds the ability to make a whole new plant. This means the future plant must have the start in life with all the minerals, vitamins, enzymes, lecithin and natural oils it needs to make trees, bark, limbs, leaves, stem, fruit and materials to bear again to carry on its own kingdom. The very nutrients contained in plants that give them their procreative ability can also be used by man to get all the procreative material necessary for reproduction, gland energy and brain components. Man must have seed materials to reproduce his kingdom.

Whole foods have been put together by nature and it's very difficult for science to see how everything is put together. They have tried to duplicate chlorophyll; they have tried to duplicate vitamin E and many of our other vitamins, but they do only part of the job. When laboratory materials have been used on live animals and plant life, we don't get the same results as we do in using the natural things. This has been proven by making vitamin A acetates, for instance, which are laboratory made, and it will never compare to the natural vitamin A as found in beta carotene, carrots and green foods.

The whole foods have been put together in such a way that we must recognize all the things that go into making these whole foods. This is why the tree is considered the sinless symbol in all our biblical history. We can make crippled trees and crippled plants when we do not have the proper elements.

Dr. Albrecht at the University of Missouri, did much work on fertility, etc., and showed that the plant life molds to the kind of soil in which we plant. The weather can make changes in plant life. Most everyone's had the experience of trying to grow plant life in a dark room. They have to have light. We've even made artificial light to represent the sun and to compare to the sun's rays in order to have proper evaluation in the plant life when it is grown indoors.

I spent time with Dr. John Ott of Chicago, who did a lot of work with color. His work showed that when he put in plastic windows instead of glass, this allowed the ultraviolet light to enter. Glass permits only 20% of the ultraviolet sun rays. His 18-year-old arthritic dog recovered and got his joint activity back again after being allowed to receive the sun's rays through the plastic windows. Even his procreative ability was there again.

It is a strange thing to see how the sunshine itself is an important part of our life. The fresh air is an important part of our life also; these work together. Did you know that 85% of the tree life in Los Angeles County has been destroyed, broken down or distorted by the gases in the air? Yes, there are so many problems we have to overcome. One of the main things we have to understand about whole foods is that they go through a filtering process, taking the most soluble trace minerals, being the most colloidal in traveling ability going through fiber structure and tissue structure—whether in a plant or human being—and in that filtered material, it can become part of the plant. We are missing the finer forces in nature that brought this whole food to us, and it can bring us the whole health we need.

I strongly advise you to read my book **The Tree of Life**, to be released soon. You are that "tree of life," and you will get a lesson again that shows you why the tree is that symbol, free of all sin and one that is fed by a stream of life we also have to find ourselves in, or we cannot be in the best of health.

Whole Foods

Tomatoes	Radishes	Celery
Broccoli	Peppers	Kumquat
Cauliflower	Lychee	Loquat
Orange, seeds	Mango	Passion fruit
Peach	Pear	Banana
Plantain	Asparagus	Prune
Beets, greens	Alfalfa sprouts	Brussels sprouts
Cabbages	Carrots	Chard
Collards	Cucumber	Endive

Romaine	Leaf lettuce	Garlic
Green beans	Leeks	Onions
Kale	Chives	Mung sprouts
Lentil sprouts	Parsley	Mushrooms
Sweet potato	Parsnips	Soy sprouts
Rutabaga	Watercress	Turnips
Bamboo	Yams	Bok choi
Barley greens	Apricot & seeds	Whole grains
Cod roe	Eggs	and others

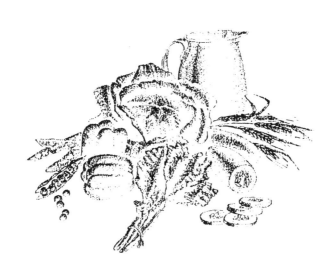

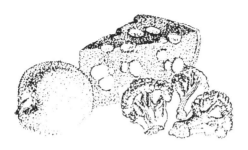

5. BRAIN AND NERVE FOODS

The brain, nervous system and the glandular system are where the greatest catalytic action takes place in the body. This is where the enzymes are necessary to bring in the greater electromagnetic forces from nature through our raw foods taken into the body.

There has to be a return to the natural foods, otherwise the spark of life that comes from the brain, nervous system and the glandular system will disappear. These organs are the ones to care for the finer forces of nature. This is where music is experienced. This is where our feelings exist. This is where we can smell the perfume. And these actions are all coming from the brain. Our five-sense organs are located in the brain. We see with the brain and the nervous system. We see and feel with our glandular system as well. The pheromones that exude from our body come from us when we are aroused from either fear or excitement. The knees, toes and hair have nothing to do with this, but the brain, nervous system and glandular system are where this "spark of life" is generated and carried on.

The brain, nervous system and glandular system have to have a certain chemical makeup, and if we are weak in these particular organs and don't feed them properly, the body just follows along and we are just existing. There is plenty going on around us in our color these days. We should know that red is an arterial stimulant; green is our greatest builder and repairman for the body; yellow is a digestion color and a joy color. Pink can be a very festive color. All the colors affect us. All natural laxatives are yellow and orange. Why? We have no training to know that the brain, nerve and glandular systems must be fed and taken care of. The same elements that feed the nerves also feeds the glands. That which feeds the glands also feeds the nerves. They are both the most sensitive parts of our body. They work in a vibratory world. All messages received by the body go through the brain first. It travels there by way of vibration, over the nerve sheath, which is very high in silicon. That's why we feed the silicon foods when we do not have the best attainment in our vibratory activity from the messages from the brain to the different organs of the body. When the organs in the body do not respond, it is possible the brain, nerve and gland system are lacking in the proper chemical elements.

Silicon is a magnetic element, and without magnetism in the body, we can't even wink and mean it. Our glandular system does not respond. We have to have the brain and nerve foods. Too many people use foods to build bone and muscle. There's too many people with just this particular expression in life. We have to have those who are concerned with the spiritual activity in life, and this is a brain faculty. We have to have those who are interested in home life and parental activities. This is evident when 40% of our children return from school to an empty house. There's no mother or father to greet them. Children are lonely, and they get almost out of hand today because they do not have the family values in the brain they should have.

We have to consider not only color, but music as well Sometimes music can be detrimental, when it is irritable to the nerves. Music has its effects, and we should study what music can do in the body. We should study what vibration can do. Vibration has a connection with the next generation, and the building up of our brain and nervous system.

We have to pick out good company, know when to rest, when to let go, learn when to relax, recognize that a busy body never repairs itself. It's only in quietness when the body can repair and rebuild itself. There are many things we should know from a brain and nerve standpoint. When we fortify the brain and nerve system with all the materials so it can exhibit itself properly in a physical way, then we have a normalcy working and nerve system with all the materials so it can exhibit itself properly in a physical way, then we have a normalcy working between the mental and physical body, and even the spiritual body we well.

An awareness can come to the person who is on the spiritual plane, and it can be a great thing. It helps him in his procreative activity the same as is working in the salmon that swims 1500 miles back to its spawning ground for reproduction. Salmon that have been created in a stream, getting ready to go to the rivers, mix with other salmon that were spawned in other streams. But when these fish are ready to spawn, they go back to the stream in which they were spawned for this particular activity. Do you think the eyes, skin, fins or scales carry the material to know this? Of course not, it's the brain and nervous system—the procreative system.

There is a sign of starvation in every disease and this lack is what we have to consider in our work. So when we have a chronic disease, we have to feed it and care for it. We have to feed sick people not only the best foods but the best of "foods" for their minds. Many people who have regained their health become new people because of what they are doing for themselves in their feeding program. This is what we are doing—feeding hungry people. Sick people are thirsting for knowledge. They want to do the right things. My average patient wants to do the right things but doesn't know what that is. An education with just a little study will help you find out the main things to do to have health and exhibit wellness.

The average person doesn't know what it is to be truly well. The medical profession tells us that 8-out-of-10 people who say they feel fine have a chronic disease. It's a sign that the brain, nerves and glandular system needs to be fed. We are not able to live a life where we can exhibit the finest.

I believe there are very few people who know what it is to really feel wonderful. I think very few people really know what it is to be well. I have never found a "well" person in my practice, which covers 65 years. The ultimate is in reaching for that perfection. It's almost like a god, a thing just ahead of us, but without these ideals or the goals to reach, we couldn't

DR. JENSEN'S

- Recommended -
Daily Food Proportion

1. Eat natural, pure, whole & fresh food.

2. 60% of everything you eat should be raw.

3. **Balance your diet.**
(80% alkaline and 20% acid)

4. **Consume in proper proportions:**
6 vegetables, 2 fruits, 1 starch and 1 protein.

5. **Eat a variety of foods everyday.**

6. **Separate starches & proteins**

7. **Include fiber.**
(Plentiful in most raw food and grains)

8. **Do not overeat.**

9. **Cook without water, high heat or air touching hot food.**

10. **Bake, broil, roast or steam your meat.**
(No more than 3 times a week... fish preferred)

11. **Use proper cooking utensils**
(Stainless steel at low heat)

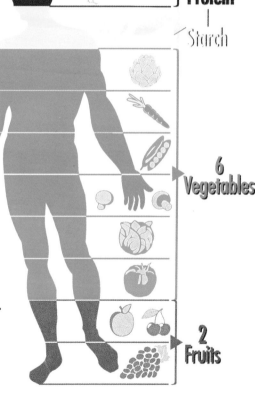

1 Protein

Starch

6 Vegetables

2 Fruits

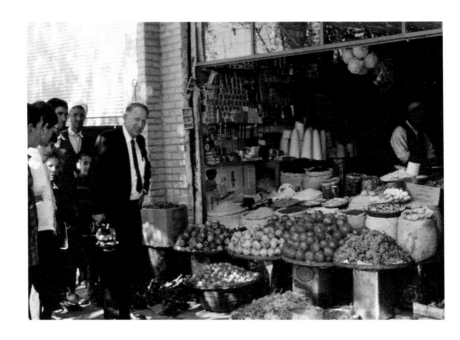

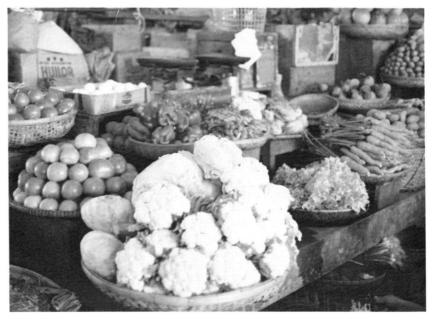

Top: A wide variety of fresh, attractive vegetables is a very good incentive to have raw foods in your diet. Bottom: Most markets in foreign countries have beautiful organically-grown fresh vegetables and fruit available quite inexpensively.

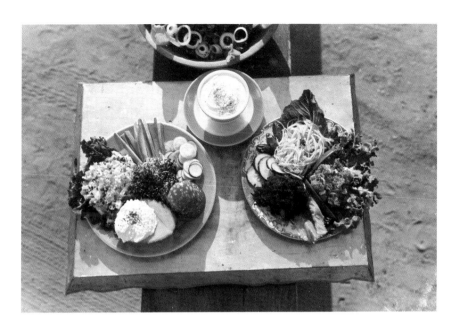

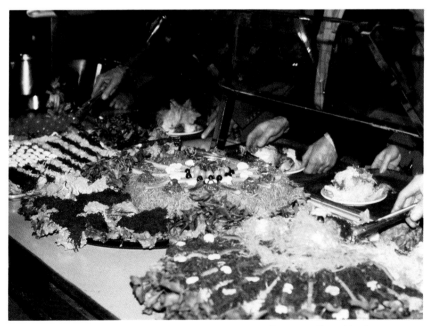

Top: Live it up with natural foods, artistically arranged. Bottom: Vegetable platters in rainbow colors were always served to patients at our Ranch.

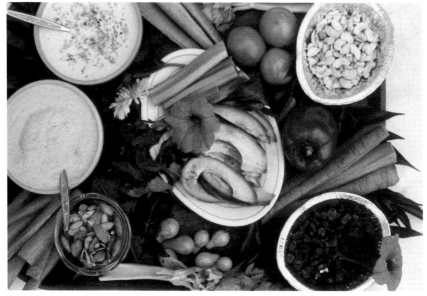

Serve your foods in an attractive manner to whet the family's appetite.

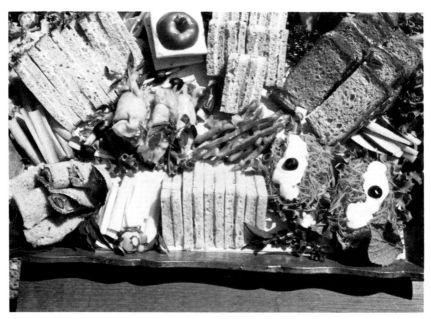

If you occasionally have sandwiches, be sure to include plenty of raw vegetables that carry water. Use whole grain breads also.

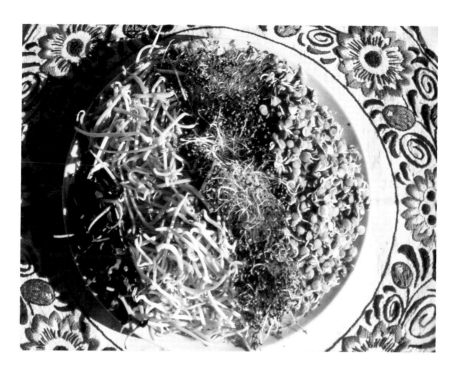

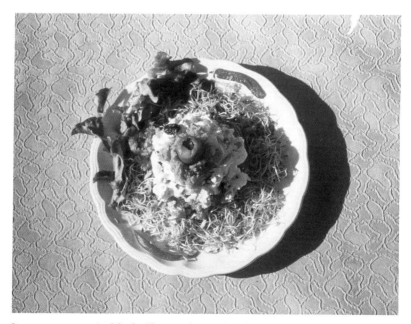

Sprouts are our survival foods. They are the most live foods we have. Include them in your diet daily to treat your body right.

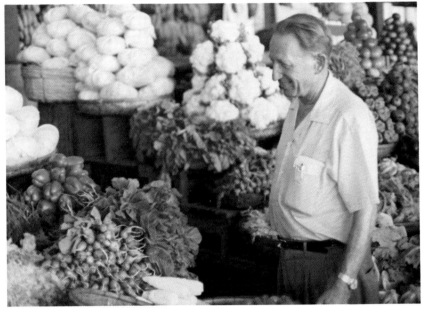

Dr. Jensen visits a fresh produce market in Japan.

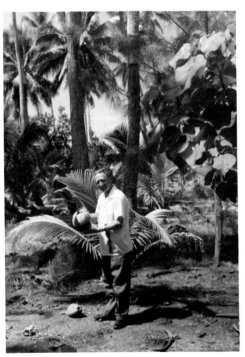

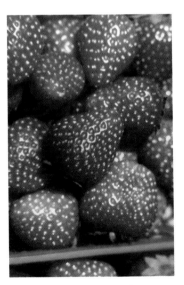

Strawberries contain the life-giving seeds and they are high in sodium.

Fresh coconut milk is a perfect protein and should be used more in the diet.

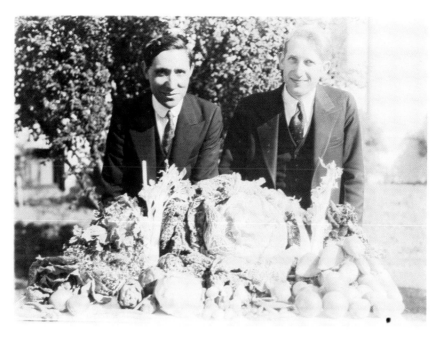

Dr. Jensen's interest in natural foods began early in his career.

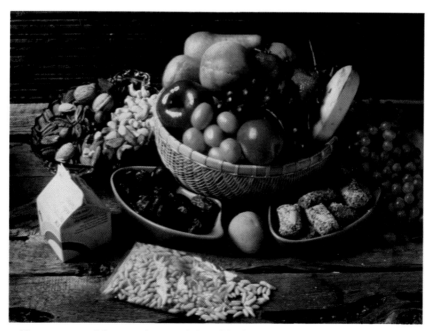

These are some of the natural, pure, whole and fresh "convenience foods," with no artificial additives.

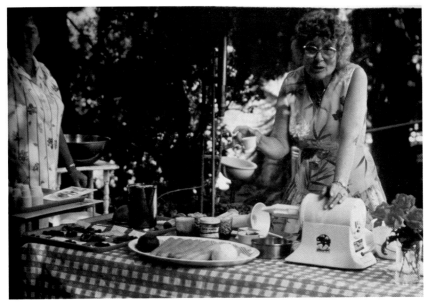

Here Marie and Sylvia demonstrate some of the methods to prepare raw vegetables.

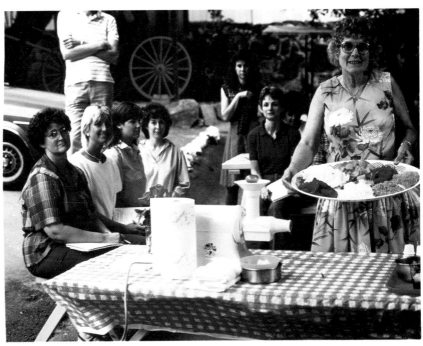

Marie with the "fruit of her labor" for a waiting hungry class.

improve our lives or our health. You can be better as you go through life. It all depends on whether you choose to live or die.

BRAIN AND NERVE FOODS

The following foods are the most important to consider in regaining your health. They are a mixture of vegetarian and nonvegetarian foods. Vegetarians may have a choice.

Gelatin	Dr. Jensen's Forever Young products	
Iodine*	Silicon*	Calcium*
Sodium*	Sulfur*	Phosphorus*
Lecithin*	Ginseng*	Ginko
Chlorella	Veal joint broth	Colostrum
Goat milk	Goat cream**	Goat butter
Goat cheese**	Egg yolk**	Cod roe***
Turtle broth	Rice bran syrup	Vitamin B*
Clam broth***	Rice polishings*	Fish soup***
Germ of grains*	Cod liver oil***	DNA & RNA*
All seeds*	Nuts (hard shell)*	Persimmons*
Shark fin soup***	Lady's slipper*	Avocado*

---

*Foods for vegans.
**Foods for lacto-ova vegetarians.
***Foods for vegetarians who eat fish.

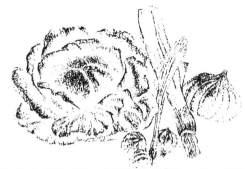

6. THE FOUR CHEMICAL ELEMENTS

There are four chemical elements I feel are missing most in practically every patient who comes to me. These are calcium, sodium, iodine and silicon. They are most prevalent in their expression and exhibition in the physical endeavors that people complain about. Each of the chemical elements mentioned here is not everything in itself. The body is a synthesis of many chemical elements and maybe a hundred trace elements. There's a lot of activity going on between these elements that we are prone to miss in life.

I studied the chemical elements, especially with my mentor, V.G. Rocine, and he taught me that the chemical elements have quite a story to tell. They are active in life; we live on them—depend on them. We belong to the dust of the earth. We're in a cycle, a temporary stage of having minerals coming and going. We have a transference of the old for the new; as we die daily, we also live daily.

We make new skin on the palms of the hands every 24-to-48 hours. We are a temporary instrument. This body has just been loaned to us. It has been put in our care so we cannot allow the boys on the street to throw stones at it. We have to pain this "house" once in a while to preserve it. We have to feed it to keep the joints active.

We have to have an exhibition of what we expect from this human body. This cannot take place unless we have the chemical elements to work with, because each of the elements has a job to do. For instance, calcium is called "the knitter." Whenever we have a broken bone to knit, when repair has to take place, we have to have calcium. There's 4-1/2 pounds of calcium in the average human body. If there is a shortage of calcium, the bones cannot knit. Every disease needs knitting. Every disease needs calcium. Every patient I've had has needed calcium. This is one of the most important elements we have. Bruising and many other things in the body come because we do not have enough calcium.

When a woman is pregnant, she needs a lot of calcium. A new bony structure is being developed in her womb, and it requires calcium to develop properly. If there isn't enough of this element furnished from the mother's regular diet, then her supply will be robbed. It will be taken from her joints, glands and every organ in her body. Back problems begin to develop because of the lack of calcium. I have very seldom seen a women who's delivered two or three children who's recuperated from the depletion of calcium. So it is well to know that calcium is probably our most important element.

There are three other elements I feel are equally as important. The next is sodium, the "youth element." Sodium keeps us young, active, limber, pliable and able to jump for joy. We're not so settled we can't move. Sodium is what keeps calcium in solution. When you go to the doctor and he says the joints are getting stiff because you're getting old, that's not entirely correct. Your joints are getting stiff because sodium is lacking in the joints. Many times people are told there's nothing you can do for this. All they offer are drug treatments to relieve your pain. Sodium is lacking in the body and we look to artificial sodium to neutralize the acids. There is a food sodium that can do a much better job. Sodium is stored in the stomach wall, joints and lymph stream mostly, and these three areas cause the most trouble in our civilization today. So sodium has a story to tell. We must feed sodium to the body.

Iodine is "the metabolizer." Every activity of every organ in the body is slowed down when the thyroid gland does not work normally. It can even bring hyperactivity into the body. But a hyperactive thyroid gland needs iodine because it is burning it out. Because of this, we begin an underactivity of the thyroid. Many times it is caused because of toxic materials. Then we have a toxic thyroid gland. When metabolism gets slower, this brings on a lowered activity in every body organ. When the hormonal values that come from the glands are not going into the body from a wellness standpoint, there may be a lack of certain hormonal values in the body. Even the bowel transit time is slowed because of the lack of proper thyroid metabolism.

Every organ is affected by the lack of proper thyroid activity. So we look now to the thyroid as a very important organ in the body. Usually the average patient I see has a lack of activity in the body organs. We try to bring up the activity to a normal state by treating the thyroid gland. I can tell you that 90% of my patients, after the age of 45-50 years—both men and women—have a lack of thyroid activity. This is why I say iodine is one of those chemical elements so necessary in getting a body well.

Silicon is called "the magnetic element." This is what I mean when I say all magnetic activities in the body need silicon. I remember years past when the radio was just coming into existence. We had a tiny silicon wire from the radio set touching a galena, and positioning it in various places would allow music to come through the earphones, but it had to be the best magnetic spot in this piece of galena. The messages in your body is somewhat on the same order. You receive messages from the brain, but the proper chemical elements must be available to receive the message. You cannot have the "music of the spheres" working through your body if you lack silicon. Silicon is necessary for messages to travel from the brain to different parts of the body.

In mentioning these four chemical elements, they are not complete, by any means, but if I can get these four chemical elements back into the body of sick people, good changes will come about. This is how we use the chemical elements to get people well.

Many times people ask why we take some of the animal products. First of all, I am a chemical boy. I have gone the aesthetic way, tried to do it all from a spiritual point, but I found my knowledge and civilization were so broken up and so lacking, that I could not find all the elements in just the vegetables, especially when the vegetables are grown as they are today.

Even the spiritual person knows that a lack of certain chemical elements will not let the spirit live in the body. We become a body without a spirit. In order to keep this body right, we have to have the proper chemical structure put together, otherwise we have no temple in which to work. The spirit is immortal thing. The mortal thing is the body. The body is only here as we take care of it and feed it. We have to take care of it through the chemicals.

We are an endangered species today because of the chemical lack in people. Even the spiritual person is not living on the wisest side of life by having vegetables in their normal form and not having the enzymes in their natural state. We're not getting all the trace minerals we need. I have to say this is very important to me to see we have the chemical structure right, otherwise, our body is not a temple of the living God. It is not a godly temple with a godly spirit.

The foods listed below are separated into the four chemical groups, and should be included in your daily diet regimen for your good health. This list is not complete, but these are the **highest** foods in each group.

Foods Highest in Calcium

Eggshell tea	Calf's foot jelly	Cottage cheese
Bone broth	Caraway	Kohlrabi
Raw cow milk	Lemons	Nettles
Cauliflower	Celery	Cabbage
Goat milk	Lettuce	Sheep milk
Kale	Sea lettuce	Curly cabbage
Black radishes	Florida oranges	Egg yolk
Raw skim milk		
Raw cheese that breaks.		
Fish with fins and scales.		

Foods Highest in Organic Sodium

Dried apples	Celery	Gizzard
Roquefort	Unpolished rice	Black radishes
Fresh apples	Beaten egg white	Collards
Romaine	Strawberries	Swiss cheese
Celery cabbage	Raw buttermilk	Swiss chard
Whole rice bran muffins		

Foods Highest in Iodine

Kelp	Bass	Quail
Nova Scotia dulse	Savoy lettuce	Sea lettuce
Silver salmon	Baked potato skin	Lettuce juice
Green turtle	Turtle broth	Raw oysters

Foods Highest in Silicon

Asparagus	Raw rice bran	Barley food
Whole rice flour	Oatmeal muffins	Celery
Alfalfa broth	Cooked whole rice	Cucumbers
Oat straw tea	Dandelion	Wild rice
Wheat straw broth	Whole rice broth	Horseradish
White onions	Strawberries	Onions
Mustard greens	Wild strawberries	Marjoram
Rice bran muffins	Steel-cut oatmeal	Parsnips

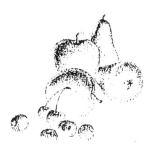

7. THE FOUR ELIMINATION CHANNELS AND THE LYMPH DRAINAGE SYSTEM

THE FOUR STAGES OF DISEASE

All diseases go through four stages: acute, subacute, chronic and degenerative. The acute stage is the active stage of disease, usually accompanied by catarrh, fever, coughing, inflammation and soreness localized in the body. Catarrh may issue from any orifice in the body such as a running nose, coughing, sneezing, tears, earwax and vaginal discharge. In the acute stage, the body is actively trying to throw out the disease, and all organs are hyperactive to support the elimination. The subacute stage is more serious. If the body fails to throw off the disease in the acute, running stage, the inflammation sinks deeper into the tissues, reducing the metabolic rate and further weakening the body. The chronic stage finds the body in a lower condition yet. This is where flu, colds and hay fever turn into asthma and occasional bouts of pneumonia. This is where joint aches turn into chronic arthritis. The final, or degenerative stage, is very nearly the point of no return. Asthma turns into emphysema. The joints swell and grow, calcium spurs appear in the arthritis case, lumps and tumors are found to be malignant.

Much of the poor health in adults can be traced back to childhood conditions. Many children's problems such as colds, flu, earaches, mumps, measles and tonsillitis should be taken care of by natural means to prevent catarrh from being driven back into the body. Cleanliness, correct foods, stimulating activities and pleasant surroundings with plenty of love will keep most children well.

THE FOUR PRIMARY ELIMINATION CHANNELS

I would like to discuss the four most important elimination channels of the body. They are the bowel, the kidneys, the lungs, the skin. The lymph system works with these four systems by serving as a "garbage collector" to carry metabolic by-products and accumulated cellular waste from tissues to the elimination organs. Each of these systems eliminates about two pounds of material per day in the normal healthy adult. If any one of these channels becomes overloaded or clogged and slowed down, there will be an accumulation of toxic material in the body tissues.

When the elimination channels have too much work to do, they become inefficient, and instead of being carried out of the body, the toxins are forced into the bloodstream and settle into those organs and tissues which have the least resistance to toxic material. These areas are usually the inherent weaknesses of the body.

The body is always generating waste material as a by-product of metabolic processes. Other waste is derived from food residues which are of no use to the body, including salt, artificial colorings and preservatives, processing by-products and other additives. Significant levels of toxins also accumulate in the body tissues as a result of environmental pollution, not only from air, water and chemicals, which are consumed or contacted directly, but also from pesticides and industrial waste which spread up through the food chain from the air, water and soil to the plants, fishes and animals that end up on our dinner plate.

The buildup of toxins in the body tissues and in the bloodstream is the pathway to lowered vitality and disease. Intestinal stasis (alimentary toxemia) in particular, is implicated in a wide range of illnesses including fatigue, headache, asthma,

hypertension, degenerative ocular changes, arthritis, degeneration of the muscles, liver, kidneys and spleen and many forms of cancer. As a result of over 65 years of work with patients in sanitarium environment as well as extensive research, I have come to the conclusion that these four elimination channels are vital to everyone's health.
Follow is an explanation of these important systems. It is important for each person to realize the necessity to clear the elimination channels, flush out the toxic settlements in the body and supply the proper nutrients.

THE BOWEL

The bowel is most important, and it is the primary organ of elimination, consisting of 20 feet of small intestine and 6 feet of large intestine. In the great majority of people, the bowel is the most underactive organ in the body. The purpose of the small intestine, with its finger-like villi, is the absorption and assimilation of foods. The large intestine is divided into four sections: the ascending, transverse, descending and sigmoid colon. It removes excess water and breaks down waste products prior to elimination. Regular bowel activity promotes health. An underactive bowel increases the burden on other elimination organs and introduces toxic material into the bloodstream and lymph system, and this material that settles in the inherently weak organs and tissues of the body. Organs most affected by bowel underactivity are the lungs and bronchioles, kidneys, skin, liver and lymph system. These organs become overloaded with toxic settlements, and this leads to underactivity and mineral deficiency. The autonomic nerve system tends to become irritated and less efficient. It should be noted, however, that a toxic bloodstream due to an underactive bowel affects **every** organ in the body. When the colon becomes toxic and clogged, many illnesses can develop.
Many have suffered from colon disorders. Studies show that over half a million people in the U.S. suffer from ulcerative

colitis or Crohn's colitis—inflammation of the colon marked by abdominal pain and diarrhea. Colorectal cancer is a serious disease that occurs in the colon or rectum. Next to lung cancer, it is the leading cause of cancer-related deaths in America. One hundred thirty thousand new cases of colon cancer are reported each year and as many as 59,000 prove to be fatal. Often celebrities are afflicted with colon troubles. The beloved Michael Landon had cancer of the liver, pancreas and colon. Raymond Burr had a tumor in the colon and underwent a four-hour surgery to have it removed. Frank Sinatra was another who has suffered with intestinal disorders, finally having to have surgery to remove a cancer. Gaylord Hauser came from Europe, and I told him he had bowel trouble and it would affect his lungs. He died a year later with pneumonia. John Wayne had lung disorders and finally the doctors discovered trouble in his bowel. James Roosevelt, the son of Franklin Delano Roosevelt, also underwent surgery for a lesion in the colon. Emperor Hirohito of Japan died from intestinal cancer. It would have been nice if all these people had known natural things that would have prevented their conditions. By taking care of inherent weaknesses before they cause trouble, one can live a happier, more productive life.

Working with our thoughts and managing our lifestyles so we have rhythm, balance and harmony are very important to having regular bowel movements. Eating our meals without stress is most important. We should take time to eat our food peacefully without television news reports that might upset our digestion. Have pleasant conversations during mealtime or eat in silence. Eat early in the evenings so you don't go to bed on a full stomach. At night the body needs to be resting, not digesting food.

Pay attention to when the bowels need to move and do not wait. Wait long enough for the bowel to empty entirely. When one ignores the needs of the bowels, they eventually interfere with the body functions. This can cause a loss of sensitivity of nerve endings in the bowel, making one unaware of its necessary functions and ultimately leading to frequent constipation. Never force or strain yourself. This could bring about ruptures, hemorrhoids or rectal problems. Varicose veins can also be caused by too much forcing and straining during a bowel movement. Another result of chronic constipation can be appendicitis. The appendix is a small finger-shaped tube that branches off the large intestine at the lower right-hand side of the abdomen. It contains a large amount of lymphoid tissue, which provides a defense against local infection. People who become afflicted with appendicitis have often been constipated for years. When the colon becomes blocked and clogged in the area of the appendix with old waste material that has not been eliminated, the appendix can easily become infected.

So the colon is the most important elimination channel for us to take care of. Many intestinal disturbances can be prevented. Eating raw or lightly-steamed vegetables and fruits is excellent for the colon. All foods that are yellow in color are particularly good for the colon. These foods are usually high in magnesium, which directly benefits the peristaltic action of the bowel. Yellow squash, yellow cornmeal and cascara sagrada (yellow in color) are wonderful foods for keeping the bowel well. Whole grains contain fibers which are like little sweepers that keep the colon clean.

I often recommend alfalfa tablets because they are high in chlorophyll and fiber to cleanse the colon, and acidophilus which puts good bacteria back into the intestinal tract. Chlorella powder and tablets are excellent foods for building and cleansing the colon. Prunes and prune juice can also be helpful in cases of constipation. Prunes have a high fiber content and contain a natural chemical which appears to stimulate intestinal contractions. Research has shown that fish oils can be beneficial in relieving bowel inflammation.

Try to avoid coffee as much as possible and teas which contain caffeine. A good substitute in the morning is a cup of warm water. Many people decide to go on the seven-day tissue cleansing program which is explained in detail in my book *Tissue Cleansing Through Bowel Management.*

Constipation can have many causes, and can lead to many other ailments. It takes time and determination to develop new eating and living habits, but for the sake of our colon health, it is well worthwhile!

Specifics for Colon Health

Foods: Papaya, liquid chlorophyll, chlorella, prunes, figs, spinach, sun-dried olives, chard, celery, kale, beet greens, whey, shredded beet, watercress, yogurt, rice bran polishings, kefir, psyllium husks.

Drinks: Parsley juice, papaya juice, chlorophyll, carrot juice, potato peeling broth, whey, prune juice, bentonite clay.

Vitamins: A, C, B-Complex, B-1, B-2, B-6, B-12, D, E, F, K, folic acid, inositol, niacin, pantothenic acid.

Minerals: Magnesium, sodium, chlorine, potassium, iron, sulfur, copper, silicon, zinc, iodine.

Herbs: Papaya, alfalfa, aloe vera, peppermint, slippery elm, cayenne, burdock, comfrey, ginger, fennel, anise, cascara sagrada.

THE KIDNEYS

There are two kidneys and they lie in the abdomen, underneath the liver on the right and the spleen on the left. They are bean-shaped organs about the size of a fist, each about 4-5 inches long and about 6 ounces in weight. The arteries that supply the kidneys arise directly from the aorta, which is the main artery of the body leading from the heart.

The kidneys are the organs that are responsible for filtering the blood and excreting excess water and waste products in the form of urine. Each kidney contains 70 miles of filtering tubules whose function is to conserve water, glucose, essential chemical elements and to eliminate acid by-products of protein metabolism and other wastes from the blood.

The kidneys filter 200 quarts of blood in 24 hours and excrete two quarts of urine. The kidneys conserve blood volume, electrolyte balance, the acid-alkaline balance of the blood and influence blood pressure and the rate of red blood cell production in the bone marrow.

Kidney disease affects millions of Americans, and underactivity is relatively common. Underactive kidneys affect the bowel, lungs, skin, lymph, heart, blood pressure, autonomic nerves and many other organs and tissues by increasing the levels of toxic acids in the bloodstream and by altering electrolyte balance. The most important waste products are generated by the breakdown of proteins. When water is lost (as the result of diarrhea or sweating), the kidneys conserve it.

Another important function of the kidneys is to regulate electrolytes and blood. The kidneys control the body's acid-base balance. When blood and body fluids become too acid or too alkaline, the urine acidity is changed by the kidneys to restore balance.

The kidneys produce various hormones which regulate the production and release of red blood cells from the bone marrow. Vitamin D is converted into an active hormonal form by the kidneys. When the body's blood pressure falls, an enzyme called rennin is released by the kidneys to act on a protein in the blood to produce a powerful constrictor of the small arteries that helps regulate blood pressure. The kidneys also excrete an adrenal hormone that acts on the tubules to promote reabsorption of sodium and the excretion of potassium.

Thus, the kidneys are very important organs of elimination, with other vital functions as well. There are a wide range of kidney disorders that affect thousands of people each year. Hypertension can be both a cause and effect of kidney damage. Glomerulonephritis occurs when the glomerular filtering units of the kidneys become inflamed. Kidney stones are usually caused by excessive concentrations of various substances such as calcium or uric acid. Infections can occur in the kidneys when there is an obstruction (such as a stone or tumor) in the flow of urine through the urinary tract leading to stagnation. Benign, as well as malignant tumors, can form in the kidneys, but these are rare.

Well-known personalities who suffered from kidney disorders were Greta Garbo, who reportedly died of kidney disease; Robert Cummings of movie and television fame, died of kidney failure also. Former Philippine President Ferdinand Marcos had kidney problems. The Boston Red Sox outfielder, Tony Conigliaro, who made home-run history by the age of 22, died of pneumonia and kidney failure. Ray Danton, a child radio star who went on to play villains and leading men in film and worked as a director in television, also died of kidney failure.

We must take care of our kidneys!

Specifics for the Kidneys

Foods: Watermelon, watermelon seed milk, pomegranate, apples, asparagus, liquid chlorophyll, parsley and green leafy vegetables. Raw juices are also excellent.

Drinks: Drink celery juice. It is high in organic sodium, which keeps calcium in solution and helps prevent kidney stones from forming. Pomegranate juice helps maintain the correct Ph balance in the kidneys to assist the kidneys in fighting infection. Parsley, black currant, beet, asparagus and grape juice (drunk separately) each help promote the healthy functioning of the kidneys. Goat whey is another drink that is excellent for the kidneys, as it is one of the highest sources of organic sodium. It is also a good source of chlorine and calcium.

Vitamins: Those particularly good for the chemical balance of the kidneys are: A, B-Complex, B-2, B-6, C, D, E, choline and pantothenic acid.

Minerals: Those important for the kidneys are calcium, potassium, manganese, magnesium, silicon, iron, sodium and chlorine.

Herbs: To balance the kidneys uses juniper berries, uva ursi, parsley, golden seal, slippery elm, dandelion, marshmallow and ginger.

THE LUNGS AND BRONCHIALS

The third elimination channel I would like to review is the lungs. The lungs are bilateral cone-shaped organs that fill most of the chest cavity. They are made up of branches (bronchioles) and clusters of air sacs (alveoli). The lungs oxygenate the blood and eliminate carbon dioxide, a breakdown product of carbonic acid in the body. The lungs are also involved in regulating temperature, acid-alkaline balance, and lymph movement. Underactivity of the lungs and bronchioles affects the bowel, kidneys, skin, lymph, heart, autonomic nerves and every other organ and tissue in the body by increasing the level of carbonic acid in the bloodstream, reducing oxygenation, increasing catarrh levels and general acidity. Lung underactivity is often associated with allergies, asthma, lymph congestion, catarrhal problems, arthritis, fatigue, acidity throughout the body and lower metabolism.

A recent article published in California's *USA Today* was titled "California, Off to Strongest Start in Setting Pace to Clean USA's Air." Do our lungs need this? Indeed they do! In just glancing over a few newspaper articles I have collected, I find 44 deaths caused by pneumonia, emphysema and asthma. Another article reports "Lung Treatment Cuts Death Rate of Preemies." Tiny babies often lack a crucial substance on the surface of their lung cells that keeps their lungs from collapsing. The new treatment is a similar substance, a bovine surfactant taken from cow's lungs and sterilized. It is given to these babies for two to three days after birth, through a breathing tube. As many as 7,000 babies have had this condition and have been treated with the bovine surfactant.

Recently Mother Teresa was placed in intensive care because of pneumonia. Bert Parks, the TV game show host and beauty pageant emcee who serenaded Miss Americas for 25 years with his trademark song, "There She Is," died of inoperable lung disease. Jim Hensen, the creator of the beloved Muppets died of a multi-organ failure brought on by complications from pneumonia. Henry Ford II, who took over his grandfather's foundering company died after a battle with pneumonia. Ralph Bellamy, the veteran actor best know for his Tony-winning stage and screen portrayal of F.D. Roosevelt in "Sunrise at Campobello," died from a long-standing lung illness. Gene Tierney, the famous movie actress, died from emphysema. Even the famous musician, Wolfgang Amadeus Mozart, died from pneumonia. Actor, Gary Merrill, who was best known for his supporting roles in the movie, "Twelve O'Clock High," died of lung cancer. These are just a few out of thousands who suffer every year with lung disorders often leading to death.

We must take care of these vital breathing organs of life! Even pregnant women should take special care of their health and eat a good diet, rich with the nutrients needed by the unborn child to build health tissues, bones and organs. Many problems can be prevented.

When the lungs are healthy, they eliminate as much as two pounds of waste materials every day. When the lungs are weak and clogged with toxins, they are not strong enough to eliminate properly. Living in an environment with a high level of air pollution or working with radioactive minerals, asbestos or eating unhealthy foods can cause lung disorders. Often an excess of phlegm and mucus occurs in the lungs which is also known as catarrh.

Catarrh is the universal symptom of imbalances in the body, indicating disease-producing processes at work. It is always the first symptom to appear and it always indicates an excess of acids and mucus being developed due to tissue inflammation. Catarrh can be caused by a deficiency of the biochemical elements in the body, an imbalance or excess of them or a toxic irritant in the body. Catarrh is derived from the Greek words *cata* (down) and *rhein* (flow)—"to flow down." It is the body's normal response to tissue inflammation, and as long as it is allowed to flow, we know the body's natural defense system is working properly. Its presence often signals the onset of a cold, flu or other elimination process, but the most common response to it is to take a drug to stop it.

Catarrh can occur in any part of the body, and since the lungs are filled with small porous grape-like air sacs called alveoli, they are good collecting places for mucus to build up. What causes catarrh to occur in the lungs? There are many reasons. When a person has been a chronic smoker for many years, the lungs become filled with the noxious substances, nicotine and tar. The body produces catarrh as a protection from the irritants that are there. In a normal body, mucus is made by goblet cells in the mucous membrane linings. This mucus lubricates and protects the sensitive tissue lining these parts of the anatomy. If germ life, foreign matter or toxic substances enter the body, they are entrapped in the sticky mucus, which is eventually excreted from the body as catarrh-flowing mucus.

Catarrh can also occur in people who have certain allergies to foods such as wheat and dairy products. When white flour, sugar and pasteurized milk are mixed together, a sticky paste is formed. A paste can also form in the body. Other processed, denatured junk foods can cause catarrh as well. If the body receives one of these foods or a combination of them on a daily basis for a long period of time, they can begin to clog the pores and cells of the weakest organs of the body.

A person who has inherited weak lungs from the onset of life and then raised on "pasty" foods and perhaps in an environment of cigarette smoke, they often begin to have frequent colds. If the colds are suppressed by well-meaning mothers by giving the child medications, the sticky catarrhal material will be pushed deeper into the tissues of the lungs along with all the germ life, foreign matter and toxic accumulations it contains. This condition can later develop into pneumonia. With antibiotics administered, the child may appear to be free from symptoms, but in fact, the catarrh has been suppressed to a deeper level of tissue in the lungs.

Many times children or adults who have suppressed symptoms of running noses and coughs and are symptom-free of these particular conditions, will still feel fatigued in their daily lives. From stages of pneumonia, the body, in its effort to free itself from the overload of catarrh and toxic material in the lungs, will develop bronchitis, asthma and finally emphysema.

Most people fail to realize the price they pay for suppressing catarrh. A cough, for example, is a natural reflex action to rid the upper bronchial tubes and lungs of catarrh. From the advertisements of some cough medications, we find they work by suppressing the cough center in the medulla of the brain, which is a center directly related to the lungs. Other drugs act to dry up catarrh in the body, inviting the development of abnormal tissue pathology wherever the dried catarrh settles.

What are the alternative ways to remedy lung diseases? In my work, I do not deal with disease at all. I work with the whole body.

Elimination of Catarrh

When neuro-optic analysis discloses biochemical deficiencies in various organs, we can make diet and nutrition basic conditions in our approach to eliminating catarrh. There are two basic steps in getting rid of catarrh, and they both work together. Cleansing the body through fasting, juices and bowel management is half of the solution. Correct nutrition is the other half. We purify the body as much as we can and we strengthen it as much as we can. This assumes that we are changing food and other habits which contribute to or aggravate the catarrhal problem, because our goal is to strengthen the body until it can eliminate toxic accumulations through the reversal process and the healing crisis.

Rearranging Process

Hering's law of cure says, "All cure starts from the head down, from the inside out and in reverse order as symptoms have first appeared." Each time we have built the body up through right nutrition, exercise, positive thinking and rest to the place where it reaches a certain level of strength, a healing crisis occurs in which suppressed symptoms of disease return and catarrh is liquefied and eliminated. Depending on how chronic or degenerative the disease has become, it may take several healing crises to eliminate the old catarrhal deposits.

I have never had a person under my care for a year or more who did not notice better health, fewer colds and higher well-being. Any who have experienced catarrhal discharges from any part of their body noticed definite improvement. Properly selected foods and herbs made a decisive difference in ridding the body of catarrh.

For taking care of the lungs or any other part of the body, a person must first achieve a clean bowel. When the bowel is clean, the other organs then have a place to dump toxic wastes. A person with lung troubles should live in a place where there is clean air. They should omit dairy products, white flour, white sugar, salt, fried foods, processed foods and alcohol from their diet. All of these can cause allergies, mucus and catarrh, which the person with lung disorders must eliminate. A thorough book to read concerning the lungs is my book called *Breathe Again Naturally*.

Specifics for the Lungs

Foods: Eat raw salads, green leafy vegetables and fruit. These foods help to cleanse the catarrhal condition from the lungs. Replace all milk products with nut and seed milks. Recipes for making these are given in this booklet. Consume grains that do not produce catarrh in the body. These are yellow

77

cornmeal, rye, millet, quinoa and brown rice. If one eats eggs, they should leave the yolk raw so the lecithin within it will not be destroyed, since lecithin is destroyed by cooking above 212 degrees F. If one eats meat, it should be organically grown and very lean. It should be baked or broiled and eaten no more than twice a week. The same holds true for fish and chicken.

Also beneficial to the lungs are: Garlic, onions, leeks, turnips, grapes, pineapple and eucalyptus honey.

Drinks: Celery/papaya juice, carrot juice, watercress/apple juice with one quarter teaspoon cream of tartar, rose hips tea, goat milk whey.

Vitamins: A, C, D, B-Complex, B-1, B-2, B-6, B-12, E, F, inositol, choline, bioflavonoids, folic acid, niacin, pangamic acid, pantothenic acid.

Herbs: Echinacea, mullein, cayenne, comfrey, coltsfoot, garlic, onions, thyme, elder flowers, peppermint, yarrow, lobelia, marshmallow.

THE SKIN

The skin is the largest organ of the body, weighing six pounds in the average adult and covering an area of two square yards. Its function is to protect the body from the environment and to eliminate some of the same toxins expelled by the kidneys. Sometimes the skin is called the "third kidney." The elastic nature of the skin is perfectly designed to guard the sensitive underlying organs or tissues against chemical or physical damage. It also protects the body against excessive sunlight or the destructive effects of harmful bacteria.

The skin is a sense organ and our major contact with the outer world. It is a mirror of our general well-being. When the skin is underactive and not eliminating properly, uric acid builds up in the body.

The skin has often been neglected in testing and remedial measures as an important channel of elimination. An example of the importance of the skin would be the way the skin works as an elimination channel for the lizard. The Gila monster eliminates entirely from the skin. Lizards live in sunny places in order to facilitate the sweating process. On a cloudy day, a lizard will have a very strong odor because the toxins are not being eliminated properly through the skin.

Likewise, it is vital for the skin of a human to eliminate two pounds of toxic material each day. When the skin is not working properly, the pores can become clogged and may be dry and scaly, with boils, pimples, acne, psoriasis and so forth. An underactive skin affects other elimination organs. When the bowel, lungs, kidneys, lymph system and digestive system are sluggish, many toxins are then forced to be eliminated through the skin.

There are a variety of skin disorders, including acne, warts, psoriasis, eczema and skin cancer. Localized rashes may appear on the skin from exposure to chemicals such as paint thinners or insecticides. A rash can also appear when the body is attempting to rid itself of poisons it has held in the tissues. It is important to keep these areas clean. Stay away from chemicals and allow fresh air to get to the affected areas. Most of these conditions can be relieved through a diet that will assist the body in cleansing the tissues and replenishing the nutrients that are deficient.

Specifics for the Skin

Foods: A person should eat plenty of fresh fruits and vegetables land avoid greasy foods. Foods that have been found to be specifically beneficial to the skin are raw goat milk, black bass, rye, avocados, sea vegetables, whey, apples, cucumbers, millet, rice polishings, rice bran, rice bran syrup and sprouts.

Drinks: Raw juices that are good for the skin are a combination of carrot, celery and lemon, and a combination of cucumber, endive and pineapple.

Vitamins: Pantothenic acid, PABA, C, A, B-Complex,

B-1, B-2, B-6, B-12, E, F, K, biotin, choline, folic acid, niacin, bioflavonoids.

Minerals: Silicon, calcium, fluorine, iron, phosphorus, potassium, sodium, sulfur, iodine, copper, manganese, zinc, magnesium.

Herbs: Excellent herbs are oat straw, horsetail, shave grass, comfrey, aloe vera, burdock.

The most important chemical elements for the skin are silicon and organic sodium. Silicon helps to keep the skin supple and elastic and sodium helps to keep it soft and free from psoriasis and other types of scaling and flaking. These two elements are included in the foods and herbs that were mentioned with high concentrations of silicon being found in raw goat milk, black bass, oat straw tea and horsetail tea. Sodium is found high in raw goat milk, whey and celery juice.

Skin brushing is an excellent way to clean healthy or unhealthy skin. Brushing the skin daily helps it to rid itself of excess oils, dead skin cells and toxic materials being expelled through the pores. Calendula ointment is made from the marigold plant and is helpful in all types of bacterial or fungal infections of the skin around the mouth or region of the anus and itching rashes. Small cracks in the skin, such as splits, chapping and fissures that often occur on the lips, in the corners of the eyelids, on finger or on nipples will usually heal quickly when massaged with calendula cream.

THE LYMPHATIC DRAINAGE SYSTEM:
THE CLEANSING RIVER OF LIFE

The lymphatic system is a network of vessels that drain lymph fluid and carry it centrally throughout the body then it eventually reenters the bloodstream. It is part of the immune system and plays a major role in the body's defenses against infection and cancer. The lymph fluid is a very clear, thin fluid that is almost like a gas and composed of about 80% sodium.

There are 45 pints of lymph as compared to about 14 pints of blood in the body of the average adult. The lymph carries nutrients to the parts of the body where the blood cannot go and carries away wastes, emptying it into the bloodstream.

I would like to make an analogy here that helps to explain the way the lymphatic system works. When we had our Ranch, we had a drainage sewer system. If it ever got clogged and backed up, we found we had serious trouble in our cesspool. Besides that, we had a wonderful little stream going through the middle part of the Ranch that carried off excess water as well as always circulating the water, keeping it clean. Stagnant water always brought mosquitos and infestation. When it was running with clean, pure water, one could almost drink from it and depend on it being pure water at any time. However, there was a dairy farm next door with cow manure, urine and everything else that had drainage down through the fields, which sometimes would enter our stream. Our beautiful pure stream became dirty, discolored and infested with a lot of waste material that the other farm was throwing off. In other words, our stream, which was at one time pure, no longer had that purity as it had in the beginning.

I compare our lymph stream to that stream of water running through our Ranch because the lymph stream is supposed to be pure when it travels throughout the body to the various tissues. This system includes tissue such as tonsils, appendix, spleen, breast and thymus. Lymph is very important because it circulates in the joints, the lens of the eyes and other tissues not penetrated by the blood. Lymph is moved through its vessels by muscle activity, exercise and breathing. Lymph system underactivity most often affects the tonsils, appendix, breasts, joints, autonomic nerves and the elimination organs.

A major factor contributing to lymph system underactivity is weakness in the elimination organs. Infections of the tonsils and appendix are common. Unlike the blood, which has the heart as its pump, the lymph must be moved by body movement. When the lymph stream is not pure, the impurity will finally get to the joints and various parts of the body in the form of uric acid and catarrh, which can cause rheumatic problems or it can carry toxic waste from the bowel to the other tissues in the body causing toxemia, infections, aches and pains.

If the proper chemical elements are not delivered to the tissues, problems can occur. For instance, calcium is held in solution by sodium and when there is not enough sodium, the calcium will come out of solution. When this happens in the vertebrae and joints, knobs will develop. Without exercise, the lymph cannot efficiently carry nutrients to the areas where they need to go. Lymph nodes are located along the lymph stream in the joints, armpits, neck, spine and groin, where they are protected by the bony structure which is the strongest structure of the body. They are concentrated in these areas because these are the areas where the most amount of movement takes place. The nodes filter lymph fluid and remove dangerous impurities such as dead red blood cells, millions of debris-laden white blood cells, chemicals and dyes.

The lymph nodes in the lungs of people who live in large smog-laden cities are often completely black from the soot that they filter from the air. Sometimes the lymph nodes swell because of an overload of catarrh and bacteria and can be quite painful. Some people have an inherently weak lymph system. They are the ones who have "swollen glands" quite often. These people hold water in their tissues more easily than others and will display a puffiness in their face, hands and feet. They may gain weight from water retention and have difficulty losing it.

The lymph must be kept clean and free flowing like the stream at my Ranch. When it is not kept clean, wastes build up in the body and proper chemical elements do not reach the glands. Many of us are exposed to chemicals in our water and air such as fluorine, cadmium, lead, mercury, gases from automobiles and sulfur dioxides that are coming from the fumes of the oil wells that have been burning in Kuwait for over a year. All this material can slowly become part of our lung structures, and it must be eliminated in order to keep our lymph stream clean.

Boils and pimples appear on the skin when the lymph is overloaded with toxins. The skin becomes underactive. An excess amount of catarrh will begin to be discharged from the body. It flows through the nose, vaginal tract, ears, tonsils and appendix. Women can develop lumps in their breasts when the lymph nodes become clogged in that area. The lymphatic system is our most important drainage system. Lymph drainage is probably the most neglected body function in the healing arts today.

In many cases, the lymph drainage is suppressed by drugs and it backs up in the body. Never stop a discharge. There is much a person can do to prevent lymphatic congestion. When one walks, they should walk quickly, taking in deep breaths and swinging the arms to squeeze the lymph nodes. A mini-trampoline also known as a rebounder provides excellent exercise for the lymph stream. Skin brushing is also an excellent way to move the lymph.

A person with a congested lymphatic system should eliminate all wheat and dairy products from their diet. These foods become quite pasty in the body and can easily clog the lymphatic system.

Specifics for the Lymphatic System

Foods: Eat green leafy vegetables, watercress, celery, okra and apples. Chlorophyll is very cleansing for the lymphatic system. Watercress acts as a natural diuretic and assists the lymph in getting rid of excess fluids.

Drinks: Potato peeling broth and raw celery juice are high in sodium which is necessary for nourishing the lymph system. Also good are blue violet tea, parsley juice, carrot juice and apple juice.

Vitamins: Vitamins important to the lymphatic system are A, C, choline, B-Complex, B-1, B-2, B-6, biotin, pantothenic acid and folic acid.

Minerals: Minerals that are necessary are sodium, potassium and chlorine.

Herbs: Herbs that can be helpful to the lymphatic system are blue violet, chaparral, burdock, echinacea, golden seal, cayenne and mullein.

Exercises: The rebounder is excellent for moving the lymph. Walking, swimming, dancing, hiking, skin brushing and the slant board are all excellent for the lymph movement. Active exercise squeezes the lymph nodes.

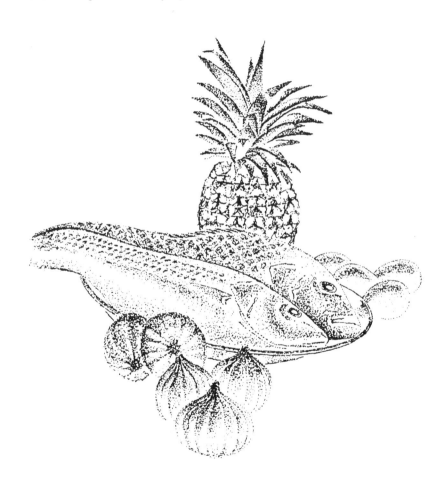

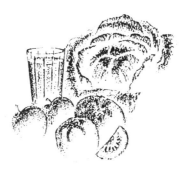

8. PHYSICAL EXERCISE

Exercise of the human body is essential to maintain optimum health. Sedentary lifestyle results in the loss of muscle mass, tone, flexibility, strength and vitality. In addition, there is a loss in similar qualities for tendon, ligament and bone. Other tissues tend to atrophy, which leads to physical degeneration.

All nutrients are assimilated better when we exercise regularly. Heat generated by physical exercise is a crucial regulator of many bodily functions. Some of these include the burning up of toxins, the removal of gaseous waste as a result of cellular metabolism, enrichment of blood with vital oxygen, the improvement of nerve communication and function, the increase of the number and size of blood vessels, the improvement of blood circulation and more.

If all other health-building practices are followed, and exercise is neglected, you will not have the best of health. Physically-active people are generally more alert, happy, cheerful, helpful and vital.

Walking or swimming half an hour daily provides the best all-around exercise. The legs must be used, because they are the pumps that drive the venous blood back to the heart.

PHYSICAL CONSIDERATIONS

- Slanting board exercises daily to strengthen abdominal muscles and bowel tone.
- Rebounder exercises 15 minutes daily to music. Increase to 30 minutes over one month's time.
- Sunbaths to promote vitamin D production. Expose body to sun daily 10 minutes per front and back (20 minutes total). Best time is between 10 am and 11 am.
- Exercise of some kind is essential for your well-being. Rebounder (mini-trampoline), running, walking, swimming, bicycling, tennis, hiking, etc., on a daily basis for a minimum of 30 minutes. Work up a sweat and breathe deeply.
- Periodic spinal adjustments for delivering ultimate nerve force to the body, such as chiropractic or osteopathic adjustments.

SLANT BOARD EXERCISES

The slant board is one of the finest and simplest pieces of exercise equipment for helping deal with any condition due to gravity, pressure or stress of daily life. It can be used for such symptoms as conditions in the bowel, a dropped transverse colon, senility (by getting blood back to the brain), brain anemia, fatigue, varicose veins, hemorrhoids and so on. The slant board helps compensate for the pull of gravity on the various organs of the body.

In every fatigue and tired body, the transverse colon begins to drop. The transverse colon is made up of the softest tissue in the body. It is tied up on the extreme right side and on the extreme left side to ligaments that go to the spine. I believe that 8-out-of-10 people who have back troubles have a prolapsus that is basically the root of their troubles, by causing a pulling on the lower part of the back. The slanting board helps correct this.

Further, the slanting board helps relieve the pressure of all the upper abdominal organs that have dropped and rested on the lower abdominal organs such as the prostate, uterus, rectum and bladder. A good deal of prolapse problems in the abdomen can result in hemorrhoids.

SPECIAL NOTE FOR SLANT BOARD USERS

Certain individuals should not use the slant board. Anyone suffering from a degenerative disease with tendency to bleeding should avoid the slant board. Instances of internal bleeding, high blood pressure, extreme obesity and easy fainting, when the head is below the rest of the body, are among those conditions contra-indicating the use of the slant board. Pregnant women should also avoid the slanting board. If you have any doubts or hesitations about using the slant board, check with your doctor.

SUGGESTED EXERCISES ON THE SLANT BOARD

Always wait two hours after eating before using the slant board.

Follow instructions for the exercises below carefully. You can feel relaxed, refreshed and invigorated quickly by stimulating circulation to all parts of the body. Do not try to do too much at first. Take on more exercises gradually. Do not attempt exercises that might endanger a physical condition. (See *Special Note for Slant Board Users* above.)

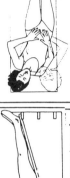

2. While lying flat on back, stretch the abdomen by putting arms above head. Bring arms above head 10 to 15 times. This stretches the abdominal muscles and pulls the abdomen down toward the shoulders.

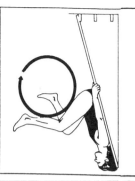

4. Pat abdomen vigorously with open hands. Lean to one side then to the other, patting the stretched side. Pat 10 to 15 times on each side. Bring the body to a sitting position, using the abdominal muscles. Return to lying position. Do this 3 to 4 times, if possible. Do only if doctor orders.

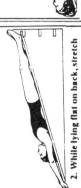

3. Bring abdominal organs toward shoulders while holding breath. Move the organs back and forth by drawing them upward, contracting abdominal muscles, then allowing them to go back to a relaxed position. Do this 10 to 15 times.

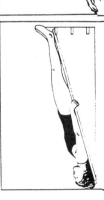

1. Lie full length, allowing gravity to help the abdominal organs into their position. Lie on board at least 10 minutes.

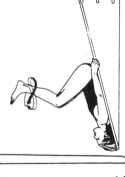

8. Bicycle legs in air 15 to 25 times.

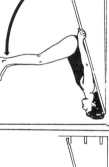

7. Bring legs straight up to a vertical position and lower them to the board slowly. Repeat 3 or 4 times.

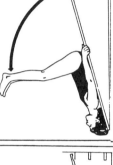

6. Lift legs to vertical position, rotate outward in circles 8 or 10 times. Increase to 25 times after a week or two of exercising.

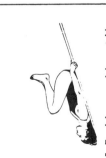

5. Bend knees and legs at hips. While in this position: (a) turn head from side to side 5 or 6 times; (b) lift head slightly and rotate in circles 3 or 4 times.

EXERCISING TO MUSIC

When doing any kind of exercises, one way to "lift the burden" is to have lovely music playing, especially the waltz. Researchers have found that the rhythm of the waltz: one, two, three (pause) one, two three (pause), is the closest to the heartbeat and we actually gain energy by listening to the waltz. Other rhythms, especially heavy rock music seem to drain energy in the long run.

REBOUNDER EXERCISES

Since aerobic exercises began growing in popularity a number of years ago, indoor bouncing devices like small, short-legged trampolines have become available. Some are round, some are square, but all of them combine fun, convenience and wonderful vitality-building exercises. The great advantage of these bouncers over jogging or running is that they are springy and do not put such a jolt on the spine. They can be used rain or shine, and as often as you like during the day.

The legs are the pumps that drive the venous blood back to the heart, and the rebounder provides a wonderful way for working the legs to move the blood into all parts of the body, as well as exercising the heart and lungs. Air is drawn deeply into the lung structure, bringing a rich supply of oxygen to the blood cells which are pumped throughout the circulatory system. This raises the vital energy at the cell level and rids the body of carbonic acid and carbon dioxide wastes. Using the rebounder is an excellent way to oxygenate the blood, improve circulation, exercise the heart and lungs and get rid of metabolic wastes.

The lymph system, vital to health, is a network of vessels in the body very much like the blood circulatory system, excepting that it has no heart to act as a pump for it. Exercise is the only way we move lymph throughout the body, since it is only through muscle contractions that the lymph is "squeezed" along through its vessels. The lymph is prevented from flowing backward by numerous one-way valves. To show the importance of lymph fluid, we have three times as much of it in our body as we do blood.

What does the lymph fluid do? It serves many functions, but its most important role may be as a key part of the body's natural immune system. Lymph nodes at the knees, groin, elbow, armpit and under the jawbone make lymphocytes, which consume bacteria or foreign matter that gets past the neutrophils. Plasma proteins that form antibodies are also made in the lymph nodes. So, we see one of the primary functions of the lymph system is to carry off toxic wastes, and we must keep it moving to get the job done. We must exercise to have a healthy lymph system and we must have a healthy lymph system to have a healthy body. The lymph also functions to bring nutrients to the cells and to carry away metabolic wastes.

The spleen is the largest lymphatic organ in the body. Others are tonsils, adenoids, appendix and breast tissue. The spleen acts as a garbage collector for worn-out red blood cells and other debris, while the tonsils sometimes pick up so much toxic material they become swollen and inflamed. If the lymph is not kept moving, toxic-laden areas can become sources of infection and inflammation.

The rebounder is one of the best ways to keep the lymph stream moving and avoid health problems.

The skin is sometimes called the "third kidney," due to its role in elimination, and, when we exercise, the heat produced by the body increases the rate at which carbonic acid, waste salts and water are eliminated through the skin. Using the rebounder is a convenient way to work up a light, healthy perspiration, getting rid of toxins and cleansing the skin pores.

Some have claimed the rebounder is a great help in losing weight, while others claim benefits to the eyes, particularly, if certain eye exercises are followed while doing the body exercises.

So, considering all the advantages of the rebounder in terms of benefits to the lungs, heart, blood and lymph circulation, waste elimination, weight control, stress reduction and possible improvement of vision, it is obvious that this marvelous miniature trampoline is one of the most versatile and health-enhancing pieces of exercise equipment we are likely to find.

OTHER BODY EXERCISES

There are other "exercises" that stimulate the body in different ways, and I consider these exercises extremely important for the health and well-being of everyone.

Skin Brushing for a Special Glow. The skin eliminates two pounds of toxic waste each day. These uric acid crystals, catarrh and various other acids are more easily eliminated when the top layer of dead skin is removed. The skin helps get rid of uric acid to relieve the work of the kidneys, which normally get rid of two pounds of waste daily.

I believe that clothing helps make us vulnerable to many diseases. It is important to realize we have to compensate for wearing clothing and other unfavorable habits sanctioned by society. Clothes keep our skin from "breathing" properly. We do not allow our body to perspire in the fresh air often enough. We do not allow the sunlight to reach the body through air baths and sunbaths. To compensate for these shortcomings that cause inactive skin, a major eliminative channel, I recommend skin brushing. Also, clothing is not, in itself, the only problem for the skin—it's the kind of clothing we wear. All synthetic fabrics: nylon clothing, pantyhose, etc., keep us from perspiring properly. Cotton and other natural fabrics absorb toxins and waste material from the skin. Synthetic materials block this elimination.

A **natural bristle** brush with a long handle should be used for skin brushing. **Never** use nylon, which will irritate the skin. Always brush dry skin, not wet, for 2 or 3 minutes each morning before a bath or shower or before dressing for the day. Rotate brush in all directions, avoiding the face. (A special soft brush may be obtained for the face.)

Kneipp Baths. The Kneipp bath is a wonderful water treatment for better circulation in the legs. It also relieves heart pressure. The bath consists of splashing through a 25-to-30-foot walk in cold water up to the knees, then a barefoot walk in grass or sand until you are dry. Do not wipe dry; if you do, you lose the value of the bath. The value is in warming your own circulation and working to make sure the circulation takes care of the effects from the cold water. This exercise builds up the resistance in the body to take care of ordinary problems.

Another way of taking the Kneipp bath is with a common garden hose, without the sprinkler attachment. Run cold water, starting at the farthest point from the heart, which would be the ankle of the right leg, move the water in a stream from the toes to the groin, then around and down the back of the leg to the ankle. Spray first the right leg front and back, two or three times; then do the left leg in the same manner. You should be able to count to six while running water up and down each leg.

This exercise is very good for circulation of the entire body. Again, don't dry off. Run or walk until you are dry and warm. Do this exercise at least once a day.

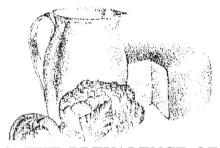

9. THE PREVALENCE OF MENTAL AND PHYSICAL CONDITIONS LEADING TO VARIOUS DYSFUNCTIONS IN THE BODY

We must always consider that diseases come slowly. We might develop a traumatic mental disturbance from years of worry or stress, and over time, this wears on the nervous system and produces nerve depletion. When we are constantly feeling rushed and have fear and worry in our daily routine, we disturb the adrenal glands. In the old days when people had tremendous fear of a wild animal, the adrenal glands pumped adrenaline to give the body energy for "fight or flight," and people used this adrenaline by either fighting or fleeing. Now when people are under tremendous stress, the body still produces adrenaline, but often their feelings are internalized. They neither fight nor flee from the situation. In a business, people become stressed with work or their boss. In school, students become stressed by time limits and examinations. At home, spouses become stressed with each other or demanding routines with their children. Anger, stress and fear are often held in for years. Whatever is not "expressed" becomes "depressed."

Many mental and physical health practitioners today are recognizing that often mental and emotional conditions are having a direct effect on physical disorders. Research is showing that hormones produced daily over years of time from unhappy emotional feelings can disrupt a body's physical balance and lead to disease. A stressed body which does not get enough rest will be much more susceptible to periodic colds and flu. Stress directly affects the immune system.

After years of sanitarium work with thousands of patients, I began to notice patterns in my patients who had emotional disturbances and how their ways of thinking and lifestyles had affected their health. I began to search for a better understanding of the links between emotional, mental and physical health. Where should we start with all of these deficiencies that are developing in the body? How long is the period of time before mental disturbances begin to show physically? How should we look at them? How long does it take for water to drip onto a stone until it is washed away? It is hard to believe that it can take 20 years to start cancer in the body. How long does it take for emotional strain to break down a physical part of our body?

I have discovered that it's a matter of getting back to how we think and how we take care of our emotional feelings. We should ask ourselves, "Are we happy? Is our life flowing in rhythm, balance and harmony? What can we do to create a healthy, happy life? Have we looked at the beauty of a flower lately? Have we been able to slow down properly? Have we been able to feel the warmth of the wind or a cold breeze that may cause a tingle in our toes? Are we aware that the mental and emotional life are probably the most important things to take care of?

When we deal with the brain, we have to recognize that it is a physical organ. This physical organ depends on what flows through it. We can have a godly attitude, a happy attitude, a deceitful attitude, a fearful attitude and these attitudes will have a direct effect on the type of hormones the brain will produce and send to different parts of the body. You will feel this in your step and even in the marrow of your bones. It has been said so many times that God can only do for you what He can do through you. If you are blocked in your attitude with fears and doubts about life, then it is much more difficult to allow loving feelings to flow through. We can do much for our attitude by working with our internal thoughts and by rearranging our lifestyles.

My whole life has been based on finding a good healthy philosophy to live by. Without a good philosophy, a person cannot be well. There are two axioms I learned years ago that I am very much in agreement with. One is, "We live on what we pour out." The other is, "I don't feel sorry for the man who dies; I feel sorry for the man who does not live well." It isn't really how long we live, but how well we live while we are living! My mother used to say that you could lose all of your money and you've lost a lot; if you lose your health, you've lost still more, but if you lose your peace of mind, you have lost everything!

In evaluating the many different people who have come to me, I look over the mental substances they work with and call it a part of their living habits. I find that many have developed nerve rings and nerve depletion. They have broken down the chemical storage houses in their bodies; namely, lecithin, phosphorus, vitamin E and vitamin B. These mental and nerve substances are so usable in our daily mental activities that we should know, first of all, how to stop breaking down.

There are many symptoms, and all doctors know the importance of mind over matter. We control ourselves and organize our lives through the mind and the brain. One out of every seven people in the USA are taking tranquilizers. Many people make a living on selling tranquilizers. More money was earned on the sale of valium one year than on all the automobile sales put together.

In the following table, I have listed the prevalence of chronic dysfunctions, as I have found them, based on the thousands of patients I have worked with and observed.

PREVALENCE OF CHRONIC PHYSICAL DYSFUNCTION AMONG DR. JENSEN'S PATIENTS

Eliminative Systems:

Bowel	100%
Skin	100%
Kidney	100%
Bronchi/Lung	100%
Excessive Transit time	100%
Hemorrhoids	100%

Circulatory System:

Circulatory Impairment	80%
Anemia in Extremities	80%
Arcus Senilis	85%
Venous Congestion	50%
Poor Oxygenation	50%
Anemia	85%
Hardening of Arteries	30%

Glandular:

Low Thyroid (over 45 yrs)	80%
Adrenal Deficiency	75%

Structural:

Stress	65%
Fatigue (tired tissues)	95%
Lower Back	75%
Poor Posture	40%
Hardened Joints	50%
Fingernail Complaints	60%
Rough Skin/Hair Problems	75%

Toxemia:

Drug Settlements	100%
Petrochemicals	50%

Nutritional:

Low Nutrient Density	100%
Lack Dietetic Knowledge	100%
Lack four most important elements: Ca, Si, Io, Na	90%
Lack Knowledge of Risks of Wheat, Milk, Sugar, Fats, Oils, and Salt	85%
Dietary Lack of Proportion, Variety, Fiber, Raw Foods, Combinations;	
Overeating	85%

WHOLISM

We hear much about the wholistic healing arts these days, and this has come about because no one has a disease of one organ while the rest of the body is healthy. We have contributing factors, trigger symptoms, reflex activities where the organ is poor, function is diminished and the hormone or enzyme activity is depreciated. Whenever this happens, in any one organ, it affects every other organ.

Many times we do not treat the organ we should. The four elimination channels, I believe, produce more troubles with other organs. If you look at the prevalence percentages in the body that develop over a period of years to make a full-blown disease (which may not come for another 20 years), we should start making changes early. We should start before a complete deficiency has developed in the various inherent weaknesses of the body. Start before clinical tests prove it to be serious. If we start early, before the ultimate breakdown, before one bad organ affects other organs, before we get into degenerative stages, then we can deal with the whole body, work with the wholistic healing arts to set up a proper lifestyle to produce the highest well-being possible.

Some of the symptoms that can indicate that the body needs help include: sweating hands, gritting teeth, nose picking, bruising easily, dry skin, brittle nails, joint stiffness, bad breath, bowel bloating, constipation, dizziness, menstrual dysfunctions; and there are hundreds more. This means there may be ten to fifteen organs to care for. This has to come from proper nutrition and supplying needed chemical elements. In your body's maintenance program, check which symptoms you may be experiencing from the following table. There is a cause behind every one. Consult your doctor or nutritionist for the elimination of these symptoms. It's later than you think!

PREVALENCE OF EMOTIONAL, NEGATIVE, AND HARSH
MENTAL FUNCTIONS FOUND IN OUR PATIENTS

Mental Condition	Prevalence in Patients	Mental Condition	Prevalence in Patients
Anxiety	50%	Lying	25%
Grief	20%	Greed	35%
Sadness	25%	Selfishness	35%
Disharmony	35%	Tempo	40%
Impatience	40%	Agony	40%
Competitiveness	30%	Misery	45%
Envy	30%	Spite	20%
Cruelty	25%	Hate	30%
Brutality	25%	Terror	35%
Stubbornness	25%	Mourning	20%
Resistance	25%	Sorrow	25%
The Executive's Dilemma:		Fear	35%
serious critical, analytical,		Jealousy	25%
exact	30%	Forgetfulness	25%
		People Problems	50%

These are faculties that people often think they need for success, but I have found they can break down the nervous system by 25% in the patients I have seen.

A HEALTHY MIND

I believe that it's impossible to be well without having a good philosophy. We have to know what it is to do the things we love to do, to eat nutritious foods, to get enough rest. We have to learn how to take on problems. It's not the problems that cause us the trouble, it's how we look at them. We do not know how to go in the opposite direction when a serious negative thing comes into our lives. We hold on to it. We often hold grudges for weeks. We get involved in the past and carry it on into the future, spoiling every moment we go through.

In all my years of working with people, I have to tell you that you can't make it if you don't have enough love. Love is the key to life and happiness, but it must be a love that passeth all understanding, a deep love beyond the physical realm. This love will carry you through and your five senses will be "fed" the proper nourishment through that love. It has a powerful effect on the physical body.

It's not just food that heals us, it's the mental and emotional aspects of our lives that make us who we are.

In order to heal yourself, you must become acquainted with Mother Earth, Brother Sun, Sister Moon and our Father in heaven. We are a part of it all. Know who you are and learn where your place is. Be good to yourself. Let there be peace on Earth and let it begin with me.

These are the emotions that can get us into trouble:

Grief	Sadness	Disharmony
Impatience	Competition	Envy
Cruelty	Brutality	Stubbornness
Resistance	Seriousness	Criticalness
Analyticalness	Exactness	Lying
Temper	Greed	Selfishness
Agony	Misery	Spite
Hate	Terror	Fear
Mourning	Sorrow	

Let's have a "commencement exercise:"
Begin to begin...a new day
Leave the past behind...where it belongs
Out with the old...to make room for the new
A new way...a better way
Let's begin with a new mental outlook
    a new physical outlook
    a new spiritual outlook.
Begin each day with a whole, pure, fresh and natural diet, outlook and lifestyle. Take time each day to know what you like and what you don't like. Guide your life in the direction that's right for you. Be the captain of your ship.

Learn how healthy foods come from organic soil and grow from the ground up. Learn about the Kingdom of Man and the Kingdom of God and work with these kingdoms to build a healthy mental and physical body. We are mechanical, chemical, emotional, mental and spiritual human beings. We must work with the plant kingdom, the animal kingdom, the water kingdom and all that dwells therein. We can develop our senses to a higher attunement to enjoy the vibrations of the sun, earth, air, colors, sights and sounds. We can become responsible for our Earth and realize that we are doing into a new planetary millennium in which we must become conscious of recycling and working with nature.

LET'S STOP BREAKING DOWN

Nutrition, what we eat, is so important for nourishing the brain, nervous system and entire body. When our brains and nervous systems are fed the foods they need, we can be stronger physically as well as emotionally. This is something to think about. The brain and nervous system are physical structures that have physical needs. When they are not receiving the proper nutrients, we could become tired or even depressed.

To heal ourselves emotionally, physically and spiritually, we must change our thoughts to be more positive. At the same time, we should change our foods to those of the highest quality to feed our brain, nervous system, bones, muscles, skin, internal organs and entire body.

Many people think they are eating nutritious foods, but often they are eating the same thing every day. To get all of the nutrients our bodies need, we have to have a variety. Very few people eat whole nourishing foods with a nutritional food plan that will ensure variety in their daily diet. If we eat the same foods day after day, week after week, year after year, we are bound to have deficits of vitamins and minerals. This can make a person ill or chemically imbalanced.

It has been my experience, after 65 years of working in the health field, that when a person gets the proper nutrients from a variety of different whole organic foods, thinks happy thoughts and lives a harmonious life, their body will grow strong and healthy. Our bodies have a great capacity to heal themselves when given the environment and nutrients they need. It's also important to eat foods that are in season. These foods are ripened on the vine in the natural sunshine and are much more nutritious than those that are grown by unnatural means when it is not the season for them. Our bodies can also create allergies when they are given the same foods over and over. Nature provides seasonal foods so we can rotate what we eat. For example, tomatoes are in season and ready to eat in the summer while pumpkins and many of the squashes are ripe in the fall. We should become aware and work with Mother Nature. She provides us with so many different nourishing fruits, vegetables, nuts, seeds and grains.

It has been my quest throughout all my travels around to world to endeavor to put together a food plan that would ensure variety and a wide spectrum of foods that would supply the fiber, vitamins, minerals and enzymes a person needs. I recommend the following nutritional guide to be followed daily, unless you are on the tissue cleansing program: 6 vegetables, 2 fruits, 1 starch and 1 protein. Sixty percent of these foods should be eaten raw. This is to ensure that we get enough fiber and living enzymes that are so valuable for digestion. Also we should never heat oils. This changes the chemical matrix within the oils and causes them to be harmful to our bodies. Cold pressed oils are better and should be used, without heating, occasionally in salads. Cook in stainless steel, low-heat cooking utensils. Never fry foods. Always use fresh, nature, pure, whole organic foods.

I tell my patients and students there are five nutritional "sins" that can cause problems if we eat a lot of them on a regular basis. These are: wheat, milk, sugar, fat and salt. When used in excess, these items can cause an overload to our systems and create catarrh, mucus and even allergies. Of course, the more harmful things are: caffeine, cigarettes, alcohol and drugs. If you want to be healthy, these things must be omitted entirely.

It is important to realize that lowering our fat intake by 3% causes a 10% lowering of blood cholesterol. (When we cook fatty foods in which cholesterol is initially balanced by lecithin, in the raw, uncooked state, using heat over 212 degrees F., we destroy the lecithin, leaving only the cholesterol. If the cholesterol had been balanced by lecithin, it would not be deposited on arterial walls.)

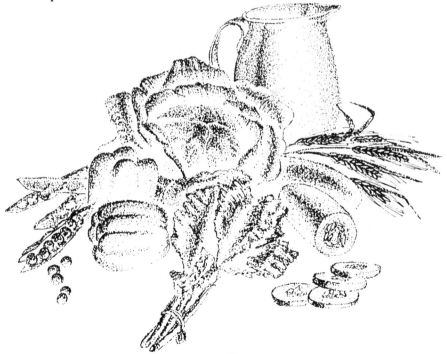

JACOB RINSE SUPPLEMENT

From near death due to cardiovascular disease, the chemist, Jacob Rinse, recovered his health enough to resume chopping wood and riding his bicycle 10 miles or so daily. He gave much credit to the following combination of nutrients, taken at the same time:

Lecithin	5 gm
Vitamin C	500 mg
Sunflower seeds	12 gm
Vitamin E	100 I.U.
Brewer's yeast	5 gm
Vitamin B-6	40 mg
Bone meal	2 gm
Magnesium	100 mg
Wheat germ	5 gm
Zinc	10 mg

In 1980, over 25 million Americans were past 65 years of age. When the body's efficiency is diminished as shown in the chart below, the processes that contribute to disease must be countered by a balanced diet and supplement regimen, regular exercise, a healthful lifestyle, a cheerful disposition and tissue cleansing (as described in my book *Tissue Cleansing Through Bowel Management*). To prevent disease and ailments, we must compensate as much as possible for metabolic slowdown associated with aging.

BODY CHANGES WITH AGING					
Age	Muscle Strength	Lung Capacity	Blood Cholesterol	Maximum Heart Rate	Kidney Function
25	100%	100%	198	100%	100%
45	90%	82%	221	94%	88%
65	75%	62%	224	87%	78%
85	55%	50%	206	81%	69%

Figures were taken from "Newsweek Magazine," March 5, 1990.

Be kind to yourself. Realize how important each and every human life is and that you are one of them. Recognize how the mind and body work together and that we are much more than the physical alone. We are physical, mental, emotional and spiritual beings. All parts of us need to be nourished—the physical brain with healthy foods, the emotional, mental brain with healthy thoughts. Organize your life in such a way that you can be happy and healthy.

If this seems overwhelming at first, begin with something small like using whole, raw foods instead of denatured canned foods. Drink herbal teas or coffee substitutes instead of caffeinated beverages like coffee, tea and cola. Caffeine is very damaging to the nervous system, emotional system, physical body and brain. It can make you think you have lots of energy when your body could actually be exhausted and need rest.

Breathe more deeply, relax, find some time each day for yourself. When you have stress, find out what the source is and try to work it through. Perhaps we don't have to "fight or flee," but we just need to have a good talk with our spouse, friend or boss. Perhaps we need to get a bicycle and ride it at the end of a hectic day at the office. Find what it is you need, and do it! Realize that what you do today is paving the way for all of your tomorrows and, like a baby learning to walk, we must begin with the first step.

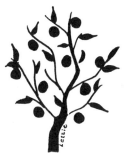

10. THE REVERSAL PROCESS

When the health level improves as the result of changing to a right way of living, all tissues and organs cooperate in strengthening the weaker tissues in which suppressed materials have been stored. The stored toxic materials begin to be activated, moistened, liquefied again, as if the body was being reversed to a previous condition of illness or disease. This is actually what happens in the reversal process. Sometimes we bring back our old problems because, as we have built up our body toward disease, there has to be a return toward good health, passing through old symptoms as we progress.

As we develop new tissue in place of the old, we go through the reversal process, which is nature's way of cleansing and restoring the body. We call this replacement therapy—new tissue in place of the old that is not satisfactory. When we reverse the process that brought on a disturbance or disease, we will eventually liquefy and eliminate the old toxic material and catarrh from the body, and the conditions which brought on the problem will be eliminated. *New tissue grows in place of the old.* This is true healing, and it is nature's way because tissue is restored with full recovery of function and activity.

HERING'S LAW AND THE REVERSAL PROCESS

Hering's law says, *All cure comes from the head down, from within out, and in the reverse order as symptoms first appeared.* This is a homeopathic law of cure. I use this as the basis for getting my patients well.

This law means that as we follow the path of good health, every organ and tissue in the body begins to be strengthened and renewed. The stronger ones support the inherently weak tissues until a point is reached where the healing powers within eliminate the stored-up catarrh, toxic material, old drug residues and pollutants. Health is worked for; it is earned and it is learned!

THE HEALING CRISIS

When we begin to eliminate old material, we have reached what is called a "healing crisis." This is the crowning reward of our efforts, a spontaneous and natural cleansing.

Unlike a "disease crisis," in which symptoms show that a toxic acid condition is developing in the body and the body is coping with the development of a disease, a healing crisis shows that old toxins are leaving, never to return if a person continues living right. Yet, it resembles in every way a disease crisis, except that it lasts only a short period of time. The healing crisis is the return of a problem from the past.

Old Symptoms Return. There may be singly or in combination such discomforts as vomiting, diarrhea, fever, rash, skin eruptions, discharges from any or all orifice of the body, for about three days. Then it is gone, and the body is much cleaner. You will feel wonderful. This is nature's way of cleansing and healing.

During the healing crisis, you should rest as much as possible, taking only a little broth, vegetable juice or chlorophyll and water now and then. This healing crisis comes when we follow the right nutritional way and the new lifestyle path.

The main way to distinguish between a *disease crisis* and a *healing crisis* is that a healing crisis usually comes at a time when you have never felt better. One day you are walking on

"Cloud 9," and the next, you are flat on your back, feeling miserable. This is usually a healing crisis.

This is an organized system. It's no "fly-by-night" idea. This works and everyone who follows this program will find out that it works. We have used it on thousands of patients, and those who have gone through a cleansing and purifying process have developed these healing crises. Patients have eliminated some of their oldest health problems and many are now living in the best of health.

If the disease has gone too far and nature hasn't the ability to bring a return, then there is only one other way to turn, and that is conventional medicine, hospitals, drugs, surgery, etc., but we are trying to bring out that much can be done **before** we get to this extreme degeneration stage.

My books *Vibrant Health from Your Kitchen, The Doctor-Patient Handbook* and *Tissue Cleansing Through Bowel Management* are among the best guides to good health. These books will help you greatly in better understanding the reversal process, Hering's law of cure, the healing crisis and what you need to know to develop good food habits and a beneficial lifestyle. You will also learn to use delicious, healthy recipes.

KNOW IT TAKES ONE YEAR TO GET WELL

When a person is working to get well on a natural program, they should realize it will take approximately one year for the body to repair and regenerate. This is true healing and not just treating the symptoms.

In order to build a whole body, we need whole foods that are fresh, pure and natural. I suggest we choose the colors of foods from the colors of the rainbow. In this way, we are assured a variety of nutrients that will nourish every cell in the body. Most illnesses are the result of a deficiency in one or more of the chemical elements.

At the end of a year of getting the chemical elements necessary for health, a person will have a stronger reserve build up. A person must live through four seasons and build the body with the natural nutrients from the foods that are produced in each season. And just as we plant seeds in order for them to be harvested when they grow, we have to plant the seeds that are necessary to build good health in order to reap a harvest at the end of the "healing season."

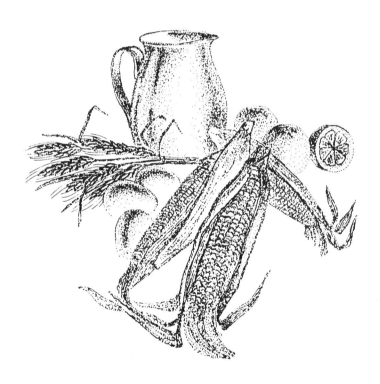

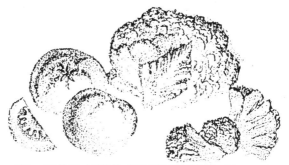

11. TODAY'S ENVIRONMENTAL PROBLEMS—WHY SUPPLEMENTS ARE NECESSARY

In today's world, there is air pollution, depleted soil, polluted waters, fruits and vegetables that have been sprayed with toxic pesticides, endangered species which are vital to our eco-systems and "holes" in our ozone layer. The amount of rich topsoil that is so necessary to provide the minerals necessary to grow our plants and thus keep us healthy, is eroding. Toxic waste dumps are accumulating around the planet giving out noxious fumes. Our immune systems are breaking down because we are eating mineral-depleted foods, breathing polluted air and drinking water that has been treated with chlorine to kill the harmful bacteria.

Are there any real and practical answers for mankind? What can be done to manage the rapidly deteriorating situation on our planet? What can one do to keep well while living in a polluted city? How does one cope? I have addressed the answers to these questions in several of my books including *Empty Harvest, Survive This Day, Soil and Immunity, Chlorella, Gem of the Orient* and *Chlorella, Jewel of the Far East.*

For people who are obliged to live in large cities, there are powerful supplemental foods they can take to ensure they get the nutritional chemical elements they need in order to stay well. Chlorella is one great example of these. Chlorella is an algae that is filled with all the vitamins and minerals needed for the health of human beings. It contains chlorophyll which plays a large role in keeping the blood clean. When the blood is not clean, then no part of the body can be truly healthy because the blood carries nutrients to every cell. Research has shown many other amazing benefits of chlorella.

At a conference on Bio-Regenerative Systems sponsored by NASA in Washington, DC, Dr. Dale W. Jenkins of the Office of Space Science and Applications had this to say: "It has been amply demonstrated that chlorella can be used in a closed ecological system to maintain animals. The algae gas exchanger has the capability of efficiently supplying all required oxygen, rapidly and effectively removing all carbon dioxide, removing excess water vapor from the air, removing toxic odors from the air, utilizing waste water from washing, recycling water to provide clean water for drinking and washing, supplying food to animals to produce animal fat and protein." Because chlorella is so efficient at transforming sunlight into biological energy, chlorella could become a good fuel source in the future. Research has shown that chlorella is a good digestant for sewage, producing methane gas and fertilizer as by-products.

Chlorella, vitamin C, COQ-10, alfalfa and vitamin E are wonderful for getting rid of the free radicals which form in the body from pollution, radiation, toxic chemicals, overexposure to the sun's rays or toxic foods. Free radicals are atoms or groups of atoms that can cause damage to our cells, causing aging, a weakened immune system and infectious diseases. These supplemental foods have a chelating ability to pull free radicals out of the body. They also nourish the body with important elements for the immune system. Acidophilus is another wonderful supplemental food that is actually a friendly bacteria that is vital to our digestive system. Acidophilus helps to fight harmful bacteria in the colon.

Echinacea is an herb that helps to rid the body of catarrh and mucus that often collects in the lungs from breathing bad air. Vitamin B-Complex nourishes the nervous system and helps one to handle the stress of the times. Calcium, magnesium, silicon and phosphorus are minerals that are important to the health of the bones, teeth, skin, hair, nervous system and are also extremely important to the proper functioning of the immune system.

People who live in cities should get a good water filter. They should buy organic foods whenever possible and eat only that which is pure, whole, fresh and natural. As often as they can, they should go to the country for exercise and fresh air. They should take moments each day for contemplation and meditation to rest their nervous systems. Thus there is much to be done to prevent disease, to keep our health and to rebuild the health of the Earth.

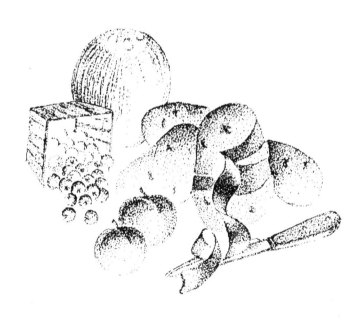

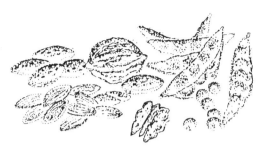

CONCLUSION

I have spent a lot of time working in the drugless healing art over the years, but I must say, there are no treatments that are worthwhile or complete without the use of nutrition. The housewife and cook are more important than doctors and specialists in the building of health and in the cure of disease. The cook can help her loved ones into an early grave with her choice of foods. It is the responsibility of each cook to know all she can about nutrition, food chemistry and food properties to keep her family well.

It is impossible to keep healthy on a wrong diet regimen. Almost all diseases are diet diseases. As long as we eat wrongly, our doctors cannot cure us. If we eat rightly, we don't have need for doctors. We have to learn how to heal ourselves. I have counseled patients, striving to guide and uplift them by building their health and teaching them that there is a right way and a wrong way to live.

In order to get well, we must exercise, cleanse and purify our bodies. I have said many times, "You can't pour new wine into old bottles." In other words, we can't have new tissues until the toxic ones have been eliminated. It is important to exchange old tissue for new, old habits for new and healthier ones. This is called replacement therapy. Replacement therapy can work in all phases of our lives. We can replace caffeinated teas with herb teas, white flour with whole grain flour, sugar with honey, fried foods with baked foods, sad friends with happy ones, negative thoughts with positive thoughts, sedentary lives with exercise, toxic water with pure water, polluted air with fresh air. Many people have lost all of their reserves and are living in a deficit. When there are no more chemical elements to sustain the tissues, they become toxic and tired.

I have helped my patients by using a combination of proper nutrition, exercise, positive thinking exercises, water treatments and other natural methods. This has been my method of treating my patients for many, many years, and it has proven to be very successful.

Despite the growing body of documented medical evidence that diet both causes and cures disease, nutritional awareness remains far from a 20th century world ideal. Only 24 of 130 medical schools in this country require future doctors to take courses in nutrition. By omitting the subject of nutrition, 80% of America's medical schools are not only perpetuating a nutritional "knowledge vacuum," they are sending out a negative message about the importance of nutrition in health as well. With our doctors ill-educated on nutrition, it's no wonder the public continues to lag in its own nutritional awareness.

The story of nutrition is not simply one of cure. It is also a story of life-enrichment and well-being. Sadly, many people are living at only 50% of their full health potential, not really sick, but not truly well either. These people need to understand that the same foods that heal by rebuilding damaged tissue will enhance wellness by increasing the efficiency and energy level of underactive endocrine glands, and all other organs, glands and tissues.

The basis for proper nutrition is found in the use of fresh, whole, pure and natural foods. The number of calories in a meal means nothing unless they come from a proper balance of foods. If there is inadequate protein, the diet can cause you to become ill. If there is inadequate vitamin and mineral content, the same may happen. Even fats, in small quantities, are necessary for metabolism. Without the proper balance of a variety of nutrient-rich foods on a continuing basis, a good health cannot be achieved and maintained.

The message, then, is clear. You **can** feel wonderful, if you will simply eat healthful foods and avoid harmful foods.

If You've Enjoyed Reading This Book . . .

Colostrum: Life's First Food—This book is full of fascinating surprises about a healing food that is "a new star on the health food horizon." It should be required reading for everyone interested in wellness and the reversal of disease. This food could be the solution to the health problems of the future.

Tissue Cleansing Through Bowel Management—Toxic-laden tissues can become a breeding ground for disease. Elimination organs, especially the bowel, must be properly taken care of. This book tells the reader how. Bowel management through a balanced nutritional program with adequate fiber in the diet and regular exercise can often do wonders. A special 7-day cleanse will bring back energy, regenerate tissues and allow good food to let nature do its healing work.

Unfoldment of the Great Within—This new book presents some of the teachings of Dr. V.G. Rocine, together with Dr. Jensen's thoughts and philosophy. In learning ease of mind, we begin to push disease out of our bodies. We should know how to start a new life and new day to become a wiser, healthier and better person.

Chlorella, Jewel of the Far East—Chlorella is a complete food. It is possibly the most thoroughly researched food of our time. One day man will learn to live in harmony with nature. Then we will see a great restoring work being done on this planet, but until that day comes, chlorella is one of the most effective foods to protect us against the toxic effects of pollution.

Herbs: Wonder Healers—Herbalism is at least 5,000 years old, and the effects of many herbs have been carefully documented, especially in China. Health is found in herbs more specifically than in all the other foods we usually purchase. More and more people are using herbs to help reverse and prevent ailments and diseases. Don't take anything for granted about herbs. Get your copy of this wonderful book; read it, and know your herbs.

Foods That Heal—In the first half of this book, Dr. Jensen focuses on the philosophy and ideas of Hippocrates, the brilliant work of Dr. V. G. Rocine, and concludes with a look at his own pioneering work in the field of nutrition. The second half is a nutritional guide to fruits and vegetables.

Juicing Therapy—Health through nature's most natural methods. How nature heals body organs and systems. Wonderful juice combination recipes. Juices for babies and children, soups, herbal green drinks, salad dressings. Special Analytical Food Guide chart.

Garlic Healing Powers—This book contains valuable information on how garlic plays such an important role as a member of the herbal kingdom. It includes garlic research, updates and uses as well as garlic recipes and other ways to enjoy garlic. You can also learn how to treat your family pets with the use of garlic.

Check at your local bookstore for information on Dr. Jensen's books and food products; if they cannot supply them, you may order directly from our office. For a *free* catalog of all his books and supplies, you may write to:

Bernard Jensen International
24360 Old Wagon Road
Escondido, CA 92027